1 in 3

Published in the United States by Cleis Press Inc., P.O. Box 8933, Pittsburgh, Pennsylvania 15221, and P.O. Box 14684, San Francisco, California 94114.

Printed in the United States.
Design: Cecilia Brunazzi
Typesetting: CaliCo Graphics
Logo art: Juana Alicia

Library of Congress Cataloging-in-Publication Data

1 in 3 : women with cancer confront an epidemic / edited by Judith Brady.
— 1st ed.
     p.   cm.
    Includes bibliographical references.
    ISBN 0-0939416-49-2 : $24.95. — ISBN 0-939416-50-6 (pbk.) : $10.95
    1. Cancer—Political aspects.   2. Women—Diseases.   3. Cancer—
Social aspects.   I. Brady, Judith, 1937-   II. Title. One in three.

RC281.W65A13   1991
362.1'9994'0082—dc20   91-20683
                                             CIP

Grateful acknowledgment is made to the following for permission to reprint previously published material: "In Response to a Promotional Ad . . ." and "Post Diagnosis" by Sandra Steingraber reprinted by permission of the author from *Benchmark: Anthology of Contemporary Illinois Poets*. Urbana, IL: Stormline Press, 1988. "The Generic Oncologist" and "Dracula Meets a Chemo-Poet" by Helene Davis reprinted with permission of the author from *Chemo-Poet and Other Poems*, Alice James Books, Cambridge, MA, 1989. Selections from *A Burst Of Light* by Audre Lorde reprinted with permission of the publisher, Firebrand Books, Ithaca, New York, 1988. "Images of Dying" by Barbara Rosenblum appears in slightly different form in *Cancer in Two Voices* by Sandra Butler and Barbara Rosenblum, 1991, Spinsters Book Co., available from Spinsters, P.O. Box 410687, San Francisco, CA 94141. Used by permission.

1 in 3:

WOMEN
with
CANCER
confront an
EPIDEMIC

edited by JUDITH BRADY

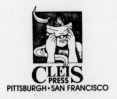

CLEIS
PRESS
PITTSBURGH · SAN FRANCISCO

Acknowledgments

I always read the acknowledgments in books. It's been comforting, I think, to know that hardly ever do people really write or put together books all by themselves. This book—more than most, I would guess—owes its existence to many.

First, of course, are the women who wrote for it. They stuck to their deadlines and were patient with my requests for editorial changes. Each woman had the courage to speak from her own experience with cancer. That takes guts. Each woman had the consciousness to look at her own experience against the background of the world in which we live. That takes imagination. Guts and imagination together are a tough combination to beat.

1 in 3 was inspired by conversations between Claude Delventhal and Cleis editor Frédérique Delacoste. Had Debra Connors not begun the work of editing this project, I would never have dared to even think about it. Felice Newman and Frédérique Delacoste of Cleis Press were willing to take a chance on me and then gave me inspiration and assistance way beyond their professional obligation. My sister, Joan Brady, showed me ways to do things when I got stuck. And then there are all the people who helped me, encouraged me, listened to my worries, and added their suggestions: June Casey, Cita Cook, Linda John, Pat Hendricks, Monika Hudson, Sharon Martinas, Bryan Nichols, Jean Pauline, David Peichert, Judy Revord, Ines Rieder, Jackie Winnow.

As the reader will see by the many references to her, no book by women about cancer can go by without recognizing the contribution made to us all by Audre Lorde. She has been a source of knowledge, inspiration, and strength to women with cancer for many years.

Finally, there are my two daughters: Maia, who cared for me when I had to battle my own cancer; and Tanya, who bore with me as I worked on this book. I love them very much.

Contents

III. Surviving the Cure: Dealing with the Medical Profession

IV. Living in Our Bodies

Introduction

There was no history of breast cancer in my family. Several years ago, during my search for something to explain why I had breast cancer, I went to the office of the National Association of Radiation Survivors. They had just moved and their files were still in packing cases, still piled up, floor to ceiling. The only other person there was a young guy off in a corner with a computer, cataloging the contents of the boxes; he told me to take a look at Box 327, which was buried deep in one of the piles. We dug it out, and I sat on the floor and spread the contents of the box around me.

The first item I picked out to look at was a photocopy of a book published in Washington in 1980 by the prestigious National Research Council; its title was *The Effects on Populations of Exposure to Low Levels of Ionizing Radiation*. The first sentence of the section on breast cancer read, "The female breast is one of the organs most susceptible to radiation carcinogenesis."

Before 1945—before the atomic bombs were dropped on Japan—breast cancer was rare among women in Hiroshima and Nagasaki. When the National Research Council did its study, some thirty years later, breast cancer was not rare at all; it was common, terrifyingly so. But I've never even visited Japan. I was born and brought up in California. I've lived in California all my life.

Still sitting on the floor, I found another study. In the first pages of this one there was a map of the United States which showed the distribution of nuclear energy and fuel production plants, weapons production and research plants, and toxic dumps—all heavy producers of ionizing radiation. What this map showed was that in California—in my state—there are more of these places than anywhere else west of the Rocky Mountains.

I sat motionless for a long time, feeling the weight of these two books on my lap and listening to my heartbeat. Then I wrote out a check and joined the National Association of Radiation Survivors. I was one of them, and I knew it.

Since 1971, when President Nixon first declared the war on cancer, the United States has spent one trillion dollars—a sum nearly a third as large as the national debt—on cancer research and treatment. Despite this money, the number of cases and the number of deaths from the disease rise inexorably every year.

My own case was diagnosed in 1980; at that time the statistics indicated that one in fourteen women in the United States would be diagnosed with breast cancer. Five years later, the figures were one in ten. Six years after that—now, in 1991—the figures are one in nine. And it's not just breast cancer. At the turn of the century, cancer of all kinds accounted for only a twentieth of the total deaths in the United States. Now it's the second biggest killer of all, and one in every three of us is going to have to face some form of it at some time in our lives.

Heredity and smoking play an important part, but these two elements alone can't explain the ferocity of what's happening now. These days babies are born with compromised immune systems; they have dioxin and a veritable arsenal of other chemicals stored in their bodies before they even take their first breath. The breast milk they drink—produced in that tissue which so readily responds to ionizing radiation—is full of alien substances. Children eat food laden with pesticides and chemical additives. They breathe car exhaust. They live in the shadow of nuclear plants and dumps. When they grow up, they work in or near those plants and dumps and in plastics factories and other places that expose them to carcinogens, known and unknown. The United States is a dangerous place to live.

When we had a country without this kind of pollution, the cancer rate was low; with this kind of pollution, the cancer rate is high. Nobody denies the correlation. Or rather, nobody denies it as long as what we talk about is comfortably remote—as long as it is statistics, charts and abstracts. When it comes to individual cases, the situation is altogether different. Let's consider the case of Millie Smith of Olympia, Washington, downwind of the million curies of radiation that Hanford let loose. She has thyroid cancer. Maybe her doctor asked her whether she smokes and whether anyone in her family has had cancer. But nobody—not her doctor, no official of the state—nobody at all will ask how long she's lived downwind of Hanford and if she was there during the years of radiation emissions. And there is Simi Litvak, who has breast cancer. She was asked about her family history, too, but no one will even bother to find out that she lived near Rocky Flats, Colorado when there was a plutonium spill. Or Karen Hopkins, who carries within her genes the imprint of her father's exposure.

There are millions like Millie and Simi and Karen. And me. And this is to say nothing of the medical response we meet or the personal reaction to the diagnosis and treatment, much of which is documented in these pages.

I have confined the testimony in these pages to women simply because I am a woman and my experience has been with women. But the questions belong to everybody. And the point of this testimony is to present the questions not in terms of abstract numbers and technicians in white coats, but in the words of the victims of the disease itself.

Judith Brady
San Francisco 1991

I. The Politics of Cancer in Women's Lives

The Appointed Day

SUSAN EISENBERG

Tomorrow I will dial the phone:
  hear it ring and be
answered, state my business
be put on hold.

My doctor will be buzzed:
decide to use the phone in his office
settle into the comfortable chair
perhaps take hard candy from the bowl.

He will reach for the file labeled with my name:
spread it open on his desk
pick up the receiver
and tell me
        yes,
        or, no

All today I rehearse tomorrow, one o'clock:
                dialing the phone
                the ring
                stating my business calmly
months of waiting narrowing toward a few
screaming moments

No, he will say
or, yes.

The Goose and the Golden Egg

JUDITH BRADY

Cancer: it's a terrible word. The very thought of cancer gives rise in nearly all of us to fear and loathing. It is a sinister thing that grows and consumes, mutilates and kills.

I have cancer of the breast. In the United States, breast cancer is the leading killer of women between the ages of thirty-five and forty-five. Now, near the end of the twentieth century, statistics indicate that one out of nine women will develop breast cancer,[1] and that *one out of three* Americans will face some form of cancer. Of these, two out of three will die from the disease. It is not a nice death.

I was forty-three years old on the morning when I discovered my cancer. My husband of nearly twenty years had recently left me, and I was still staggering from the shame of the rejection and the new, draining struggle of surviving as a woman alone with two teenage children. I awoke one Saturday morning, still groggy from the past week of work and worry, and as I pulled myself out of bed I caught a glimpse of my naked body in the mirror. I gazed sleepily at the image of my body, thinking nothing. Stretching my arms up over my head, I watched my reflection, I remember, as I slowly ran my left hand down the length of my right arm, feeling the muscles and sinews pulled taut beneath my fingers. Raising my left arm up toward the ceiling, I let the fingers of my right hand languorously caress it, exploring the curves and valleys of bone and flesh. When my fingers reached my left armpit, I felt it. I moved closer to the mirror, and as I pressed near the strange hardness I could see it—a slight, rigid swelling underneath the short dark growth of new hair. A lump.

That morning, now a decade ago, was the start of yet another battle for me. In all my attempts to anticipate and forestall disaster as I wrestled daily with a host of new fears, I had not thought of this one. Cancer—if it crossed my mind at all—was something that happened to someone else. Today, after a bilateral mastectomy, a year of chemotherapy, and two reconstructive surgeries, my cancer is in remission and no longer the focus of my fight to stay alive. Now it has become the core of a deep anger in me. Cancer—

still our modern metaphor for evil—is among the most terrible of unforeseen mistakes arising from the wanton search for progress and profit that has historically driven our society. Nuclear war is a disaster which looms over our future, but cancer is a disaster which is already here.

While it has been adequately demonstrated that cancer has existed for centuries and is not new to modern industrial society, the epidemic of this dreadful disease in our country today is clearly a new social phenomenon. In 1900 cancer accounted for only 4 percent of deaths in the United States, but now accounts for 22-23 percent and is the second leading cause of death,[2] and it threatens to overtake heart disease and become our biggest killer all too soon. Despite the silence shrouding the surge in cancer statistics and the seductive lures of self-blame/self-cure offered me by "New Age" doctrines, my own struggle with cancer convinced me that my disease and its treatment are yet another price paid for being born in a time and place where polluting the world is more profitable than protecting it. Multiplied many times by the suffering and deaths of the millions who become cancer patients, my experience is a tiny piece of our collective story, the story of a people who will continue to pay with our lives until we fight back.

For me, the battle which we as a people have yet to fight against cancer will come too late. I already have it. Like other individuals I know who have so far survived the ravages of this disease, I am not anxious to see more people join us. But the magnitude of the "cancer problem" in this country is staggering. Three out of four American families will have to cope with this dreadful disease. Those statistics translate into the probability that every time you take a stroll down the streets of any city in this country, nearly eight out of ten houses you pass will contain a family or living group at least one of whose members has or will have cancer. Most of that suffering could have been avoided.

According to the World Health Organization in 1964, 80 percent of cancers are caused by human-produced carcinogens.[3] Today the estimate is that 90 percent of cancers are caused by environmental toxins,[4] and as the pollution of our environment increases along with the number of cancers, it seems likely that the preventable percentage of cancers will increase also. A study made in 1984 for the Louisiana state legislature, a body not given to radical positions, concluded that "many, if not most, cancers are prevent-able."[5] If society caused it, society has the power to prevent it. But the cancer rate keeps rising.

And so do the denials, which have now become a litany so familiar we scarcely pay attention. Yet every time an "industry spokesman" or a government agency proclaims that this or that chemical is not harmful in such-and-such an amount, a warning bell has been sounded. There is no known "safe level" of exposure to any cancer-causing agent.[6] You can't be a little bit pregnant, and you can't be "safely" exposed to a little bit of a lethal poison. The notion of a "safe level" makes even less sense when it is placed in the context of our present circumstances. We are bombarded daily by many different carcinogens, and our embattled immune systems must work overtime to ward off the combined effects of so many toxins. Further, those overworked immune systems must carry out their tasks in a weakened condition. There is some evidence that our immune systems themselves are so severely taxed by the constant exposure to environmental poisons that our bodies are becoming less able to protect us from any amount of potential dangers.[7] Meanwhile, the numbers and varieties of those potential dangers are mounting.

Despite frequent industry claims to the contrary, the fact that cancers result from workplace and toxic waste exposure to carcinogens is well documented and incontestable. Industry routinely uses or produces countless powerful carcinogens. Asbestos, for example, has claimed hundreds of thousands of lives with lung and stomach cancer. Eleven million workers have been exposed directly since World War II, and nearly everyone is still exposed to "low levels" of asbestos in consumer products, public buildings, even drinking water. Vinyl chloride, a chemical component of the ubiquitous material called plastic, is a potent carcinogen causing cancer of the liver. Hundreds of thousands of workers have been exposed to vinyl chloride, and countless thousands more breathe escaped vinyl chloride in their air. Benzene, mostly produced in oil refineries, is a highly toxic chemical which causes leukemia and other systemic cancers. Half the population of the United States is exposed daily to levels of benzene higher than the "safe level" recognized by the Occupational Safety and Health Administration (OSHA).[8] The United Farmworkers Union has records of too many people—mostly children—who have cancers directly related to pesticide exposure.[9] The list of toxins could go on and on. In fact, an autopsy of a typical American citizen would turn up a veritable arsenal of chemicals which have settled and accumulated in the fatty tissue.[10] Further, we have yet to see the full devastation caused by leaks and failures of nuclear power plants. Certainly the 1986 disaster in Chernobyl will have terrible consequences manifested by the end of this century. Conservatively, as many as 250,000 cancers are now forming in human bodies across the world as a result of that one incident.[11] Possibly more than a million deaths will eventually result from the Chernobyl accident.[12] In our own country, the government-owned nuclear power plant in Hanford, Washington has released enough radiation to make it as dangerous as Chernobyl.[13] Nuclear weapons testing has added, and continues to add, many thousands of cancer victims to the list.[14]

Some large killers, like breast cancer, are not quite so easily connected with industry-produced chemical toxins. Yet the indirect link is there. In the late 1770s, a British physician noted a correlation between men who worked with coal and a very high rate of scrotal cancer. More than a century later, the chemical agent benzo(a)pyrene was isolated as the cause of those malignancies.[15] We now know that chemical is responsible for some other cancers as well. For instance, it is present in cigarette smoke. The Peralta Cancer Research Institute in Oakland, California, has conclusively linked that same chemical, benzo(a)pyrene, with breast cancer.[16] Benzo(a)pyrene is also a by-product of fossil fuel emission, and when ingested into animal tissue tends to attach itself to fat cells. There has been a documented correlation between overweight, a diet high in animal fat, and the incidence of breast cancer.

It doesn't take a particularly imaginative mind to make some connections here, even if those connections haven't been "proven." We live in a country where the major mode of transportation is the automobile. Our public transportation systems, when we have them at all, are too often deplorably inconvenient, severely limited, or simply unaffordable. Automobile manufacturers, the oil industry, and their hired handmaidens on Madison Avenue have together convinced the American public that each person deserves to own at least one car. Every commuter, who must drive to work because public transportation is not available or would take twice as long, knows the familiar sight of hundreds of other cars alongside, each containing only one person. The obvious waste of energy is enormous. And the increase in the emission of benzo(a)pyrene into the air is likewise enormous. That chemical settles on the grass upon which cattle graze as they breathe the polluted air, and the animal fat of the cattle becomes rich in benzo(a)pyrene. We also breathe the polluted air, taking in benzo(a)pyrene, and then drink milk and eat animal fat, increasing our dose of benzo(a)pyrene. Our breasts are largely fatty tissue. Perhaps breast cancer might not have become such a potent killer of women if our society had been one in which accessible and efficient public transportation (often powered by electricity) had priority over the profit-making needs of the automobile manufacturers and the oil industries.

There is a less elusive—and certainly more ironic—connection between breast cancer and a chemical produced by DuPont, the world's largest chemical company. DuPont has recently gone into the business of selling medical equipment, including X-ray film for mammogram machines. That same company has been identified by the Environmental Protection Agency as one producing a high cancer risk for emitting large amounts of butadiene from its Louisiana neoprene plant, and butadiene has been linked to breast cancer.[17]

A more ubiquitous danger lies in the indisputable relationship between the rise in breast cancer rates and the increase in exposure to low levels of ionizing radiation. Uterine and cervical cancer are also consequences of radiation exposure, the effects of which are cumulative. In fact, that connection between low-level radiation exposure and specifically female cancers has been understood and documented for some time, much of the evidence coming from studies of breast cancer incidence among women in Japan after the Hiroshima and Nagasaki atomic bombs.[18] I had chest X-rays (for tuberculosis) nearly every year until I was in my twenties, and I have lived most of my life in an area (California) which has a particularly high concentration of nuclear dumps, research and commercial reactors, and plutonium processing plants.[19] The female breast is one of the organs most susceptible to radiation carcinogenesis, and there are really no places to live in the United States where we can be shielded from hazardous exposure. Our medical/cancer establishment, however, has apparently been sheltered from exposure to this readily available information.

Many of our cancers are not so surreptitiously pumped into or dumped onto us. Some cancers are shrilly promoted. By the 1980s, most people were finally aware that there is a definite connection between lung cancer—the biggest of the cancer killers—and smoking. At first glance, the cancer risk from cigarette smoking appears to have an important difference from the hazards of exposure to other types of carcinogens; that is, we cannot stop breathing even if the air we breathe is poisonous, but surely we have the choice not to smoke.

I began smoking at the age of fourteen. Both my parents smoked. I was a middle-class child who approached adulthood in the 1950s, an era of strident conservatism and conformity. If I had become convinced in my teenage years that cutting off one of my legs would assure me the social success that was promised me by the multi-million dollar advertising campaigns of the tobacco companies, I would have begged to have my leg severed. Smoking a health risk? As a teenager, I was totally convinced that the question of health risks from smoking was no more than the tut-tuts of bluenoses who had morality qualms about smoking, and their objections, of course, only made smoking more attractive. There were, however, some studies even back then which indicated a link between lung cancer and cigarette smoking, but the medical profession and the surgeon general remained silent. The tobacco industry itself evidently recognized the possible dangers before the public became generally aware. The industry acted quickly to protect itself. For instance, an uncle of mine who was a surgeon went to work for the Tobacco Institute. My Uncle Jack was paid a hefty salary to help sell cigarettes to the American public and protect the $16 billion-per-year tobacco industry[20] by allaying any creeping fears we might have about potential dangers to our health from smoking. Oddly enough, he himself quit smoking shortly after he began working for the Tobacco Institute, where he was privy to data kept hidden from the public. While my Uncle Jack may have been more openly unethical than most physicians, he certainly never received any censure from his less opportunistic colleagues in the medical profession.

I quit smoking years ago, after I had been a heavy smoker for nearly a quarter of a century. Today, in my urban neighborhood, I still see teenage girls proudly flaunting their symbol of adulthood—the cigarette—as they saunter down the street in small groups, flirting with a future as lung cancer statistics in the dawn of the twenty-first century. Public acceptance of smoking is beginning to decline, but cigarettes are still legal. They are still promoted. Though consumption in this country has declined in the past few years, today we still smoke cigarettes in this country at the annual *per capita* rate of over 3,000, and production of cigarettes has increased by 39 billion since 1986 due to greater exportation of U.S. cigarettes abroad.[21] We are still bombarded with millions of dollars worth of advertising every year, telling us how sexy cigarettes will make us. And the cigarettes are still killers.

As the incidence of cancer rises, so too does the optimistic publicity about a "cure." Yet a cure for cancer does not seem likely in the foreseeable future. All cancers have in common the characteristic of cells which have gone biologically wild, but cancer is not one disease. It has more than a hundred different forms, each of which attacks a specific part of the body. Cancers are so unique that a pathologist looking at a biopsy of a tumor in one part of the body formed from the spread of cancer cells from a tumor in another part of the body can tell where the primary tumor is located. For instance, breast cancer which has spread to the bone is still identifiable in the bone tumor as breast cancer. The continual promise of a simple "cure for cancer" is more than misleading; it is a cruel hoax. As long as we are encouraged to focus our attention on the hollow promise of a cure, we are more likely to passively accept and pay the enormous cost of the "management" of cancer by the medical profession.

If you have cancer, nevertheless, you will go to a doctor. That doctor will offer you one or more of several orthodox treatments: surgery, radiation, and chemotherapy. Of those three, surgery has the best track record for cures.[22] But the skill of the surgeon works only on cancers which have not metastasized (spread), and many cancers are not even detectable until they have already spread. Some cancers may have begun to spread but not yet left evidence of having done so. In the case of breast cancer, for example, surgery is the first method of treatment, but all too often the cancer has already spread even though the surgeon was unable to find other tumors. Further, the disturbance caused by the surgical excision of a tumor always risks the increased spread of cancer cells. And a few cancer cells left alive in the body can spell death.

Radiation and chemotherapy, unlike surgery, have very poor "cure" rates, but like surgery also pose real dangers to the patient. Radiologists point proudly to the fact that radiation has been used successfully with 80 percent of patients with Hodgkin's disease. They are right, but Hodgkin's disease accounts for only 1 percent of cancers. Certain forms of leukemia also respond to radiation treatment, but—again—leukemia accounts for only 3 percent of cancers.[23]

Not only does radiation not have even a fair "cure" rate; it is often downright harmful. Mammograms, for instance, are loudly proclaimed as a first-line defense against incurable breast cancer, but there is some serious concern about the unregulated use of those X-rays on highly sensitive breast tissue, and there is reason to suggest that young women should resist the pressure of the medical profession to undergo periodic mammograms to test for breast cancer; mammograms might well be causing more cancers than they ever detect.[24] Further, the failure rate in detecting breast carcinomas by mammograms, which are extremely expensive, is alarmingly high. A study in England revealed that 40 percent of malignancies X-rayed were missed by the mammographies, and there have been estimates that the false-negative readings could be as high as 73 percent.[25]

Perhaps even more disturbing is the increasing evidence that the use of radiation to cure cancer can result in metastases or a second primary malignancy.[26] A difficult-to-detect condition known as pericardial metastasis (cancer spread to the lining of the heart) "often follows mantle radiation for Hodgkin's disease and chest irradiation for breast cancer."[27] Women treated with radiotherapy for Hodgkin's disease have developed breast cancers from the radiation.[28] Bone cancer in some children has been linked to both radiation and chemotherapy.[29]

Radiation has certainly been useful as a palliative in some instances. Tumors in the bone from metastatic breast cancer can be significantly reduced in size by radiation, thereby providing relief from pain. As a cancer panacea, however, radiotherapy is clearly a failure and a dangerous one. Still, the massive use of radiation goes on unabated. It doesn't make sense. Hospitals have spent billions of dollars on the massive radiation equipment. They are not about to let that investment stand idle, but must instead make that investment pay for itself and then continue to make profits. Thus the heavy use of radiation seems more closely linked to the eradication of hospital debt than to the eradication of cancer.

Chemotherapy is the third treatment for cancer offered by the medical profession. It, too, has been effective against Hodgkin's disease and leukemia. Some types of small tumors do temporarily respond to chemotherapy; it can buy time, but often the side effects make the purchased time a miserable experience. And chemotherapy, though used almost routinely, has not made a statistical dent in the big killers: cancers of the lung, colon and breast.[30] But chemotherapy is a favorite with the medical profession. It does not require expensive machinery. We are a drug-taking culture; the use of drugs for cancer is a natural. We expect it, the medical profession finds it expedient, and the pharmaceutical industry—one of the wealthiest of American industries—actively promotes it.[31] Chemotherapy treatments can cost up to $500 per treatment. I was supposed to have twenty-seven treatments.

The doctor who diagnosed my cancer said to me, after unsuccessfully trying to jab a needle into the hard mass in my left breast, "Well, it's certainly cancer. That one," pointing to my breast, "will have to come off." I completely fell apart and then looked for a second opinion. I managed to find a more sympathetic surgeon and within ten days entered a hospital. A week later I emerged with a modified radical mastectomy on my left side and a subcutaneous mastectomy (a "prophylactic" measure now considered too aggressive a procedure) on my right side. Before I left the hospital, the surgeon told me that he had made arrangements for me to see an oncologist and begin chemotherapy. To save my life it was necessary for me to have chemotherapy, I was told, because one lymph node was malignant (the lump I had found in my armpit), and it was likely that I had loose cancer cells running around in my blood stream looking for a cozy place to "colonize."

The oncologist wanted to do both radiation and a full year's worth of chemotherapy. I refused the radiation, largely because my unconventional surgeon had warned me about its ineffectiveness with breast cancer, but also because I knew that as soon as I physically could handle another surgery, I was going to begin breast reconstruction, and I did not want my skin damaged by radiation burns. My chemotherapy started a month after the surgery. I was given the maximum dose of the standard mixture of chemotherapeutic agents for breast cancer.

I had just started working at a new job when my cancer was discovered. I was afraid of taking too much time away from my work because I feared that a new clerical employee with cancer could be easily expendable, so I arranged to get my treatments in the evening. Every other Thursday evening I went to the clinic. For several months I was able to drag myself to work on Friday morning, but soon the accumulative effect of the drugs made working the day after treatment impossible. At first I went to the clinic by myself on the bus to get the chemicals shot into my body. As time went on, however, the poisons caused more and more severe reactions, and I had to try to find someone else to take me to the clinic and drive me home. And I needed someone who was brave enough to stay with me as the chemicals were slowly pushed into my veins.

The examining room was tiny. I would lie down on the table with my right arm extended. I couldn't be shot in the left arm because the surgeon had removed all the lymph nodes from that arm while searching for more cancer, and the risk of infection was too great. The nurse would come in bringing a tray which carried three small, sealed vials, several large hypodermic cases, some needles and a flexible tube. She always set the tray on the small table near my head. With mounting anxiety I would gaze at those bottles as I waited for the doctor to come and pump their contents into my body. After what seemed like a very long wait, the jovial doctor would enter, sit down, transfer the contents of one of the vials into a hypodermic case, and attach the tubing to a needle. He would begin kneading the flesh on the back of my right hand, looking for a good vein. When his fingertips had found their target, he would expertly slip the needle into the vein and then attach the hypodermic case filled with the drug to the other end of the tubing. With a slow pressure he would empty the case into my vein. When that was done, the second vial followed. The third vial, cytoxin, was the most difficult one for me because its side effects began immediately. The doctor would attach the chemicals to the end of the tube and very slowly begin pushing down the plunger. Within a few seconds I could feel a warm flush creep over my abdomen, and then I began to taste hot metal somewhere near the back of my throat.

By the time that third vial was emptied, I would start to feel the restlessness. My eyes would get very red and begin to sting and tear. My way of coping with the inevitable jitters—and with what I knew was also coming—was to keep myself heavily drugged with painkillers and sleeping pills until the worst had passed. I took the first pills before leaving the clinic so that I would be very sleepy when I got home. I would turn on the television set near my bed, and it stayed on for the next thirty-six hours. Every time I woke from the sleep of drugs I could see the television. If I was able to focus on the picture, I took more drugs. If I couldn't focus my eyes, I did not take more drugs. The television became my monitor. By the next morning I would begin to vomit, a natural physical function which has always been extremely difficult for me. It was easier if I was drugged. I would float to consciousness and feel the waves of nausea. In a fog I could make my way down the hall to the bathroom, throw up, and stumble back to my bed until I had to throw up again. By Saturday morning, thirty-six hours after the injections, I could ease up on the sleeping pills. By Sunday I could get up and resume life for another two weeks—until the next treatment.

In my heart I find it difficult to believe that chemotherapy cured me of anything, and I know that surviving that treatment for cancer was a terrible struggle. Cancer mortality rates seem to indicate that neither chemotherapy nor radiation has done much better for most other people. Yet chemotherapy and radiation are still given almost routinely as adjuvant cancer therapy following mastectomy and many other cancer surgeries. The medical profession has nothing else to offer. Both radiation and most chemotherapeutic drugs act by damaging cells which are in the process of multiplying. Cancer cells multiply at a much higher rate than normal cells, and are thus theoretically more vulnerable than normal cells. Unfortunately, some normal cells in the body are also fast multipliers, like cells in the stomach lining or in the hair follicles, accounting for some of the unpleasant side effects (nausea and hair loss). Radiation is the choice when there may be minute bits of tumor cells left in the tumor site, because radiation can be directed to a specific part of the body. Or there may be free-floating cancer cells in the blood stream, which calls for the systemic attack of chemotherapy. Sometimes both therapies are used, as the oncologist wished to do in my case. Usually, however, when radiation or chemotherapy is used to augment surgery, everybody is working in the dark. No one knows whether or not there is still cancer present. But there might be, given the grim statistical chances of recurrence.

When I underwent chemotherapy, I knew that there might be loose cancer cells in my body. I also knew that I might be cancer-free. But I was frightened enough by breast cancer mortality statistics (and my cancer had already spread to the lymph system) that I agreed to the "treatment." A decade later I am still alive and—for the moment—apparently free of cancer. I have no doubt that I am now part of those statistics used by the medical profession and pharmaceutical industries which "prove" the effectiveness of chemotherapy. Given that no one knew whether or not there were still cancer cells in my body, the medical success of my chemotherapy does seem a bit dubious. Moreover, most of the success (that is, survival) statistics are based on a five-year survival rate. Breast cancer, however, is generally considered a systemic (as opposed to localized) disease, and the five-year survival yardstick does not have much meaning because secondary tumors can take much longer than five years to materialize. Hence if I am still alive and cancer-free twenty years after my surgery, I will consider myself cured and a credit to the medical profession. But what happens to the statistics if I develop a metastasis during that time? Does anyone believe that the promulgators of the chemotherapy cure, who had included me in their five-year success statistics, will apologize for misleading us? Will they modify their earlier erroneous statistics to more accurately reflect their actual failure?

Not only does chemotherapy fail as a reliable cure for cancer, it has even caused some cancers. The medical literature is rife with reports and discussions about leukemia as a secondary malignant condition caused by chemotherapy. The use of chemotherapy is likewise blamed for some secondary solid tumors; chemotherapy for lymphoma has been responsible for secondary malignancies like cancer of the bladder.[32] Hepatitis and pneumonitis are other disasters which can follow in the wake of over-enthusiastic use of the toxic drugs. Severe bladder infections and dermatitis can occur. Patients are told that the complications are a small price to pay for the prolongation of life, despite the doctors' own evidence that chemotherapy may not help some patients at all. Postmenopausal women with breast cancer do not benefit from chemotherapy,[33] yet they constitute a substantial captive consumer group for the expensive chemicals.

While the medical profession continues to peddle enormous amounts of radiation and cytotoxic drugs, they remain irresponsibly silent regarding socially effective cancer prevention. The truly compassionate and competent physicians who feel real concern for their cancer patients do what they can with their limited resources. But regardless of any individual oncologist's dedication, in a health care-for-profit system, cancer is the goose that lays the golden egg.

The United States is the only industrialized country in the world except South Africa which does not have any form of national health protection for its citizens. Any illness, accident, or physical malfunction is a source of income for doctors and the myriad industries which surround medical care. To the credit of the medical profession, however, many times we at least stand the chance, *if* we can afford it, of being helped or cured when we visit the doctor. Old killers like pneumonia and tuberculosis, for instance, can now be cured. Increasingly sophisticated surgical techniques can fix many injuries to our bodies. But if you come to the doctor for cancer—as one out of three of us will—your chances of being fixed are not very good. Your chances of becoming poor, on the other hand, are excellent. At the average cancer treatment cost of $30,000 per person,* cancer has become the source of billions of dollars to the medical profession and all its allied industries.[34]

Hospitals are in financial trouble these days. If most cancer patients require surgery and lengthy hospital stays, we must make up a good proportion of hospital income; there are certainly enough of us to make a substantial contribution. Ten years ago, my combined surgeries alone cost my insurance company more than $12,000, and then I had to pay several thousand more out of my own pocket because the surgeon charged more than my insurance company was willing to pay. Hospital costs run anywhere from $400 and up per day—just for the use of the bed. As one out of nine women now faces breast cancer, breast cancer alone represents a tidy sum to the medical profession.

The drugs for cancer are a lucrative source of income as well,

---

* As medical costs continue to rise annually, the figures from any given year will be obsolete by the following year.

and the drug companies are always searching for a new and strong market. Methotrexate, one of the drugs I was given, was good for $5 million a year almost ten years ago. Adriamycin, one of the most toxic (and popular) drugs, netted $10 million the first year it hit the market, 1974.[35] The combined total annual worth of cancer drugs, excluding ancillary drugs like painkillers or antibiotics, in the United States is $750 million.[36] Even our tax monies go to subsidize the drug companies in the form of Congressional allocations for "research," the results of which are then patented by the drug company which received the grant.

"A cancer cure will be worth a fortune," a drug company executive said over thirty years ago.[37] And it's a fortune that they are after. Despite frequently glowing popular medical reports about progress with cancer and the current drugs used, the dismal facts about the unchanging cancer mortality rates and the failure of the celebrated "war on cancer" are readily available.[38] New avenues for revenue will have to be found, and it looks like immunology will be a principal one. Interferon, a naturally occurring substance which appeared to have anti-cancer properties, was a possible candidate. Unfortunately, it did not produce much in the way of encouraging results. Interferon's washout as a cure for cancer disappointed not only cancer patients. The drug industry had looked upon interferon as a very profitable breakthrough; it is fabulously expensive. There are other avenues under investigation, but as yet these avenues are used only as a "last resort." When orthodox methods have failed (and they continue to fail and fail), some patients who can afford it try immune therapy. The orthodox methods have one particularly difficult side effect in common: radiation and chemotherapy both damage the body's immune system. At this point, it doesn't seem surprising that immune therapies have failed. They are tried only on patients whose immune systems have been devastated. Still, there are more dollars to be made there. And recently a physician proposed in a prestigious medical journal that cancer patients themselves pay for the research in biotherapeutical cancer cures.[39] Needless to say, he did not mention how the profits would be distributed should that research yield a patentable drug.

The cancer rates and related death statistics have become the sort of facts and figures difficult to take into one's consciousness. They are just too big. It is estimated that in the state of Louisiana, for instance, cancer causes at least one death every single hour around the clock.[40] In the whole country there is a cancer death for every single minute of every single hour of every single day. It is all too easy to forget that those numbers represent real people who live real lives and feel real pain. In the face of mounting public fear, ineffectual environmental regulations, and impotent medical response to the crisis, people with cancer do what they can to fill in the void. Cancer clinics, alternative cancer therapies, cancer support groups, cancer counseling centers and cancer books abound. Faced with bewildering information and the specter of death, we who have cancer need every bit of help we can get to aid us in our struggle. Each individual must make difficult personal decisions about how he/she will fight cancer, and must do so alone. Organized society offers very little in the way of guidelines; other people's experience is all we have to go on.

Being suddenly forced to acknowledge one's mortality is a profoundly shocking experience, though the interruption in the routine momentum of our lives can be a motivation for truly positive changes. We can stop smoking. We can make dietary changes. Some people will be able to reduce stress levels, better enabling their natural physical defenses to fight the proliferation of cancer cells. The efforts of many cancer victims* to take control and heal themselves—seldom with the assistance of the medical profession and often in spite it—are a moving testimony to the strength of the human spirit and its will to survive.

Yet too many support groups and too much of the current popular literature approach the subject of cancer as if it were strictly an individual problem. Over and over again we cancer patients are scolded for our lifestyles and told that we have the power to control our disease because *we*, people with "cancer personalities," caused it. The bookshelves groan with anecdotal accounts of self-cure through something as definable as diet or as mysterious as visualization, each method acclaimed as the way to "take responsibility for your cancer." Many of the self-help cancer books have in common the unstated premise that you—the cancer victim—are a primary cause of your cancer.

* I use the term "victim" quite consciously, for I believe that we are, in fact, victims of a social crime, the crime of poisoning our environment. Many people with cancer strongly object to being termed "cancer victims" because they feel it implies a passivity that they do not wish to accept. I stand with them as a fighter for survival, but I insist that we recognize the real situation in which we find ourselves.

In our culture there are compelling ideological and psychological bases for adopting the view that "I caused my cancer." I know I will never forget how terrorized I was by the diagnosis of cancer when I first heard it. In the shadow of that memory, it does not seem unreasonable to me that people with cancer should try to find refuge in the view that they can cure themselves because they made themselves sick. The other side of that assumption, however, is the admonition that if you fail to cure your cancer, then it is you who have done something wrong. I remember what a brutal blow it was to all of us in a cancer support group to which I belonged when a young woman with metastasized breast cancer lost her fight. She had done the visualization and the physical exercises. She had modified her diet. She had adopted the positive outlook. She had completed all recommended orthodox medical treatments. She was an example and an inspiration to the rest of us. And she died. Her death caused many of us to begin reexamining our ideas about the causes and remedies of cancer.

Given that the profit motive is the driving force of our economic system, it's not surprising to hear industry clamor that cancer is caused by the cancer victim; any acceptance of liability could lead to financial disaster. The chemical industry created the American Industrial Health Council in 1978, for instance, to lobby against governmental interference in toxic pollution. They attributed the increased lung cancer rate solely to longevity and cigarette smoking,[41] thereby neatly placing the entire blame for cancer on the individual victim. Blaming the victim is a time-honored method of deflecting organized opposition and protecting a power base. Surely, however, it is not in the best interests of cancer patients to accept, let alone champion, the doctrine of individual responsibility.

In many progressive social movements of the 1960s and 1970s, people who had been victimized—by institutionalized racism, sexism, and other "isms" which serve to denigrate and keep powerless specific groupings of the population—uncovered and analyzed the ways we internalize our victimization and accept the blame ourselves. If we are poor, despised, ignored, or beaten, we are encouraged to believe it is because we have somehow failed to measure up. Our heads, as one woman once put it, are the last outpost of the enemy. That is, as long as we believe that we ourselves are at fault for our apparent shortcomings, those who profit from our docility are safe. The problem of runaway cancer is not much different from other social issues. As long as we continue to believe that we ourselves cause our cancers, then the real perpetrators of our cancer epidemic are off the hook.

That hook, if we had it, should certainly snag the decision makers in much of our industry and government. Industry, which produces and uses most of the carcinogens, is clearly not a potential ally in any effort to begin effective cancer prevention programs. Even though industry loses workers to cancer, there are always more workers, and the profits made are evidently enough to convince those in power that things should remain just as they are.

With its open ties to industry, our government will not be a willing ally in any battle against cancer, either. Elected representatives do not make their way to Capitol Hill without the money and influence supplied by industry and its financial magnates.

At first glance, The American Cancer Society (ACS) looks like one beacon of hope. When I had my mastectomies, I was visited in the hospital by a volunteer from Reach for Recovery, an American Cancer Society program in which women who have had mastectomies visit mastectomy patients after surgery, but only at the surgeon's request. I was still too stunned by the anesthesia and the surgery to be much inspired by her bright assurance that I would be fine and nobody need ever know, but I was very grateful indeed for the package supplied by the ACS which she brought me—enough dacron fluff to stuff the little nylon pockets included in the package so the pockets could fill out the bra I had worn to the hospital. I had already begun worrying about how I would look leaving the hospital with my newly flattened chest. Just having those little pockets was a tremendous relief, and no one else but the ACS supplies such things to women in hospitals who have just lost their breasts.

The American Cancer Society is the largest organization of its kind in the world, commanding the services of thousands of volunteer workers and hundreds of millions of dollars annually. Like most people, I had always thought the ACS existed to help cancer patients. The ACS does have some valuable programs like Reach for Recovery, but, in fact, only fifteen cents of every donated dollar goes to provide services for people with cancer.[42] The ACS would argue in its defense that it supports cancer research. That research, however, is focused on the still elusive "cancer cure," about which much ballyhoo and many promises are made every April when the ACS conducts its annual fund-raising drive.

An organization of such vast assets and resources could be a major force against the callous and short-sighted pollution of our environment and our bodies. Instead, the ACS—an organization which exists, as it boasts, solely on contributions from the public and is purportedly "dedicated to the fight against cancer"[43]—is a powerful collaborator in our national cancer cover-up. Any real "fight against cancer" must take the form of prevention, becoming a fight against the industrial pollution of our world and the connivance of government with industry in the cover-up of that pollution. But the American Cancer Society not only refrains from criticisms of industrial pollution, it actively participates in the numbing of the American public with comforting messages about "advancements in the treatment of cancer," "effective rehabilitation programs," and "improved diagnostic tests."[44] In spite of the preponderance of evidence that the only viable approach to combatting the cancer epidemic is through swift, strict, and comprehensive environmental controls, the ACS turns the definition of "cancer prevention" into an admonishment to visit your doctor more frequently![45] In only half a century the disease of cancer has galloped from ninth to second place in claiming the lives of American people, and the ACS impassively tells us to feel hopeful because cancer "statistics are ever more encouraging when they are adjusted to take into consideration other factors affecting life expectancy—for example, dying of heart disease . . ."[46] In this best of all possible worlds, the good news from the American Cancer Society is that cancer is not yet the primary cause of death.

The most striking deficiency of the American Cancer Society is that it allocates 85 percent of its money to projects other than services for cancer patients and provides virtually no support to realistic preventative measures. Unfortunately, the dubious fiscal priorities of the ACS are not its only transgressions which do not surface in its public image. The largest cancer organization in the world should logically be in the forefront of the environmental movement if it were truly about the business of fighting cancer. But the ACS, like any multi-million dollar business, is governed by a board of directors. And like its cousins in the rest of the corporate world, the ACS board of directors shares its members with other corporate entities. Those other businesses, haplessly, are often the very ones which produce the environmental carcinogens.[47]

To compound matters, the ACS played a pivotal role in the creation of the government's cancer agency, the National Cancer Institute (NCI), in 1973 and has increasingly taken the lead in directing NCI's programs and priorities.[48] The conservative stances regarding cancer treatment from both organizations may indeed stem from the fact that many drug company officials serve on advisory committees of the NCI. Of the three standard drugs which I took for breast cancer, for example, two were manufactured by companies which had officials formally associated with the American Cancer Society and the National Cancer Institute.[49]

The ACS and the NCI certainly appear to have serious conflicts of interest when it comes to cancer prevention and treatment, and they have traditionally taken a "don't-rock-the-boat" position whenever a controversy arises. While the ACS did significantly contribute to anti-smoking campaigns in the 1960s, its efforts in relation to smoking since then have been feeble at best (relying on voluntary controls), and the organization has yet to come up with any effective legislative programs. In a similar vein, the ACS has opposed warning patients against the cancer risk of hormone-containing drugs (such as Premarin, an estrogen replacement) on the grounds that such a warning would "interfere with the practice of medicine."[50] During the debate over the cancer risk of saccharin, the ACS sided with the saccharin manufacturers[51] despite evidence that there was a risk. They have been conspicuously silent whenever major public health legislation to regulate toxic production and waste has come before state or federal governing bodies.[52] They have certainly never been known to raise the question of cancer risk from our increasing exposure to nuclear radiation through nuclear power plant failures and nuclear weapons testing.

Unless the ACS takes an approach to fighting cancer which is radically different from their present activities, we will have to work without them in any struggle to rid our society of the poisons which are killing us. Fortunately, there are groups in this country working on environmental issues, but those groups will have to wage an uphill battle against the powerful industrial/military complexes and their short-term interests. Such battles will not be won with pennies. If the millions of dollars annually collected by the ACS were diverted to those groups and organizations which are truly working to clean up our environment and stop any further pollution, we might at least lay the basis for some improvement. One thing is certain. If we do not change our social priorities in this country, we can safely bet that cancer will indeed become the leading cause of death in the not too distant future.

The true tragedy of today's cancer plague is that so many people are suffering and dying from a disease which could have been prevented from claiming most of those lives. For those who know they have cancer and for those whose bodies harbor a yet undetected cancer, prevention will come too late. Action now, however, could make the literal life-versus-death difference for people who do not have cancer and for the generations to come. But too often people simply shrug their shoulders. The fatalism about cancer which Americans apparently feel is a sad reflection of our perceived powerlessness.

Cancer is not inevitable. It is not mysterious. And it is not a necessary by-product of industrialization, a price we must pay—as we are so often told—for our progress. When testing for carcinogenesis is done on any given number of the nearly 70,000 untested chemicals in use today (with nearly 1,000 more added to the list each year), no more than about one in one hundred proves to be cancer-causing.[53,54] Unless that testing is enforced by law (with no loophole of a permissible "safe level"), however, those one in one hundred chemicals will continue to do their dirty work. Even the hardhearted argument that testing is too expensive no longer holds water; vastly cheaper and easier testing methods have been developed.[55]

Radiation from nuclear power and nuclear weapons is another unnecessary source of cancer. Nuclear power as an absolutely essential form of energy is hotly defended by the nuclear industry. If we are to meet our constantly growing energy needs, say the nuclear buffs, we must have even more nuclear power plants. But Sweden, Denmark, and Austria have already abandoned or begun phasing out nuclear power,[56] and those countries haven't come to a standstill yet.

Untold millions of people have been exposed to dangerously high levels of radiation through the testing of nuclear weapons. The United States has so far refused to participate in a significant ban on that testing. A good portion of our national resources still go into the production of those monstrous weapons, even though it is common knowledge that enough weapons exist to blow our earth out of the solar system many times over. We still allow our national paranoia about security to serve as a rationale for these weapons. When, I wonder, will our national epidemic of cancer loom large enough to finally force a serious governmental re-examination of the insane manufacture and stockpiling of ever more weapons?

"What you don't know won't hurt you," adults sometimes said to me when I was a child asking questions that those adults did not want to answer. By the time I became an adult I knew that those grownups in my childhood had lied to me. The things I did not know often became my greatest obstacles. The unknown, as we all discover sooner or later, does not go away because it is not known or because—once told the truth—we choose to deny it. Nor will our national epidemic of cancer go away because we are shielded from the truth about its origins, its effects, and its magnitude.

Our ultimate salvation from the ravages of cancer lies not in the doctor's office nor the pharmaceutical laboratory, but in the political arena. If we should decide that we want a society which does not make one-third of its people sick with cancer, we will have no choice but to ruthlessly eliminate the causes of those cancers, ignoring threats of towering unemployment figures and economic catastrophe, and showing no more mercy to the cries of bankruptcy from the industries which must be shut down nor to the pleas of innocence from greedy government representatives than they have shown to our pain and grief.

I have a recurrent fantasy, one with which I sometimes console myself when I am feeling the most powerless and vulnerable. I take comfort from my fantasy, too, when I think about the beautiful, as yet unscarred bodies of my children, and then my pleasure in their vigorous physical health becomes overshadowed by an ominous anticipation. In my fantasy, the millions of us who have become society's cancer victims will simultaneously come out of our houses and offices and factories, and we will surge into the streets. "Enough," our voices will shout. "Enough of your poisons, enough of your death!" There are so many of us that industry and commerce stop. And we, the people with cancer, will not let it start up again until we know it can start up clean, free of the pollutants which are still creating cancers in more and more of our bodies. More than a thousand of us die every day in this country from cancer. Millions of us are suffering with it now, and millions of our children are already fated to be the future's cancer victims. Have we not endured enough?

NOTES

1. "Rise Seen in Risk of Breast Cancer," *New York Times* (National Edition), January 25, 1991, p. A-11.
2. Epstein, Samuel S., M.D., *The Politics of Cancer*, Anchor Books, Anchor Press/Doubleday, Garden City, New York, 1979, p. 11.
3. Environmental Defense Fund and Robert H. Boyle, *Malignant Neglect*, Vintage Books, New York, 1980, p. 5.
4. Epstein, p. 21.
5. *Environment and Health in Louisiana: The Cancer Problem*, Governor's Task Force on Environmental Health, Louisiana State Planning Office, March, 1984, p. 5.
6. Agran, Larry, *The Cancer Connection*, St. Martin's Press, New York, 1977, p. 33.
7. Marshall, Eliot, "Immune System Theories on Trial," *Science*, December 19, 1986, pp. 1490-1492.
8. Agran, pp. 19-155.
9. Chavez, Cesar, ed., *Food and Justice*, United Farmworkers of America, La Paz, California, Vol. 4, No., 1, January 1987, p. 2. (This particular issue is an arbitrary choice; almost any issue of this publication has similar stories.).
10. Agran, p. xiv.
11. Hawkes, Nigel, et al., *Chernobyl: The End of the Nuclear Dream*, Vintage Books, New York, 1986, p. 209.
12. Brass, Irwin D., Ph.D., "How Many Will Die from the Chernobyl Disaster?" Newsletter from Biomedical Metatechnology, Inc., Eggertsville, New York, May 5, 1986.
13. Wald, Matthew L., "Northwest Plutonium Plant Had Big Radioactive Emissions," *New York Times*, October 24, 1986.
14. Johnson, Carl J., M.D., "Cancer Incidence in Area of Radioactive Fallout Downwind from the Nevada Test Site," *Journal of the American Medical Association*, January 13, 1984, p. 230.
15. Environmental Defense Fund, p. 23.
16. Hacket, Adeline J., Ph.D., Director of Peralta Cancer Research Institute, from a lecture delivered during a training session for Reach for Recovery volunteers sponsored by the American Cancer Society, San Francisco, Spring, 1982.
17. *Greenpeace*, "Eco-Notes," Vol. 14, No. 5, September/October, 1989, p. 4.
18. National Research Council, *The Effects on Populations of Exposure to Low Levels of Ionizing Radiation*, National Academy Press, Washington, D.C., 1980, pp. 269-276.
19. Wasserman, Harvey and Norman Solomon, *Killing Our Own*, Dell Publishing Company, New York, 1982.
20. Environmental Defense Fund, p. 173.
21. "U.S. Cigarette Sales Down in 1987," *Healthcare Rights Advocate*, Richlandtown, PA, June, 1990, p. 4.
22. Moss, Ralph W., *The Cancer Syndrome*, Grove Press, Inc., New York, 1980, p. 37.

23. Agran, p. xiii.
24. Epstein, p. 485.
25. Skrabanek, Peter, "False Premises and False Promises of Breast Cancer Screening," *Lancet*, August 10, 1985, p. 316.
26. Moss, pp. 51-60.
27. Press, Oliver W., M.D., and Robert Livingston, M.D., "Management of Malignant Pericardial Effusion and Tamponade," *Journal of the American Medical Association*, February 27, 1987, p. 1088.
28. Curtis, Rochelle and John D. Boice, "Second Cancers after Radiotherapy for Hodgkin's Disease," *New England Journal of Medicine*, July 28, 1988, p. 244.
29. Koten, J.W., D.J. Der Kinderen, and W. Den Otter, "Bone Sarcomas Linked to Radiotherapy and Chemotherapy in Children," letter to the editor, *New England Journal of Medicine*, March 3, 1988, p. 581.
30. Moss, p. 53.
31. Moss, pp. 61-76.
32. Pedersen-Bjergaard, Jens, Jens Ersboll, Vivi Linda Hansen, et al., "Carcinoma of the Urinary Bladder after Treatment with Cyclophosphamide for Non-Hodgkin's Lymphoma," *New England Journal of Medicine*, April 21, 1988, pp. 1028-1031.
33. Sauter, Christine, M.D., letter in *The New England Journal of Medicine*, July 4, 1985, p. 49.
34. Epstein, p. 5.
35. Moss, p. 74.
36. Moss, Ralph W., *Cancer Industry*, Paragon House, New York, 1989, p. 92.
37. Moss, *The Cancer Syndrome*, p. 69.
38. Bailar, John E. II and Elaine M. Smith, "Progress Against Cancer?" *The New England Journal of Medicine*, May 8, 1986, pp. 1226-1232.
39. Oldham, Robert K., "Patient Funded Cancer Research," *The New England Journal of Medicine*, January 1, 1987, p. 46.
40. *Environment and Health in Louisiana*, p. 1.
41. Epstein, p. 457.
42. Epstein, p. 457.
43. Holleb, Arthur I., M.D., ed. *The American Cancer Society Cancer Book*, Doubleday and Co., Garden City, New York, 1986, p. xxii.
44. Holleb, pp. xvii-xxii.
45. Holleb, pp. 15-30.
46. Holleb, p. xvii.
47. Moss, *The Cancer Syndrome*, pp. 222-223.
48. Epstein, p. 461.
49. Moss, *The Cancer Syndrome*, 68.
50. Moss, *The Cancer Syndrome*, p. 224.
51. Moss, *The Cancer Syndrome*, p. 222.
52. Epstein, pp. 462-463.
53. Epstein, pp. 66-69.
54. *Environment and Health in Louisiana*, p. 17.
55. Agran, p. 64.
56. *Greenpeace*, "Eco-Notes," Vol. 12, No. 1, January-March, 1987, p. 4.

We All Live Downwind

SANDRA STEINGRABER

"We women, how in the dark we are about our bodies and what can happen to them. We ask in whispers in the corner at a party, on the telephone . . . what does cancer look like? Will I be all right?" [1]

"Most of us are unlikely . . . to be visited by death squads in the middle of the night, but our chances of getting some form of cancer are about one in three." [2]

Some time ago, I saw a photograph of a woman with a resolute expression holding up for the camera a hand-lettered sign that read, "We all live downwind." The accompanying article described the long history of radiation leaks at the Hanford Nuclear Weapons plant in Washington state and the elevated levels of cancer in the surrounding community. Something about that photograph and the woman's message has stayed with me. Maybe it was the way she seemed so determined to march upwind to the site of the danger, to the site of the decisions.

In the summer of 1979, between my sophomore and junior year of college and a few days after my twentieth birthday, I was diagnosed with bladder cancer. The tumor, of an intermediate stage and grade, was surgically removed by threading a fiber optic tube through the urethra, a process called cystoscopy. Biopsies of the surrounding tissue were normal; there were no signs of metastasis. I was not, therefore, confronted with a systemic disease—for the time being, anyway.

The reassurance of that present moment was traversed by the uncertainty of the prognosis. Bladder cancer, I learned, was primarily a disease of old men. The medical literature of the time had no information on young women with bladder cancer; there were no clues as to recurrence or survival rates. I was not even old enough to be represented in the epidemiological charts.

The past was as much a mystery as the future. What was the cause? Bladder cancer is considered a disease of industry and consumer habit. But I had never worked in a rubber factory, never manufactured aniline dye, never smoked or consumed artificial sweeteners. As an adoptee, my genetic and family medical history was also unknown territory (to which I am forbidden access by law) and could offer no clue, since open adoptions are a recent phenomenon. Adoption records are still closed in most states for adoptees born before 1960 (that is, for those of us now old enough to be at risk for adult cancers).

Back at college, with its safety and comfortable routines, and with no outwardly visible signs of illness or change, I began the process which Audre Lorde has called "the involuntary reorganization" of my life.[3]

For me, at twenty, this reorganizing was as unconscious as it was involuntary. I was shy and awkward anyway; feelings of panic, terror and anger isolated me at a time when I desperately needed support. To those around me I was alternately secretive and explosively confrontational about what was happening. I felt constantly misunderstood, stigmatized, without language. Bladder infections and bleeding kept me in a chronic state of physical discomfort and were reminders of my new identity. I confided in strangers but eschewed counseling for fear the word "cancer" would somehow be stamped in my transcript.

My friends reorganized themselves through their collective belief that treating me "normally" was the best strategy—even though my own sense was that I had become decidedly not normal. Eventually, there was a series of falling-outs I seemed helpless to prevent. I compulsively pursued perfect grades and the approval of professors who seemed more reliable in their loyalties.

Time, too, was reorganized. For the next five years, I returned to the hospital every third month for a cystoscopic checkup. Acutely painful, each of these procedures would trigger another round of infection. The interval between examinations approximated a semester's worth of time—one season. I learned to live out my life in these three-month segments, circumscribing my plans and goals to fit within these new, truncated boundaries. I dared not think further for fear the results of the next checkup would not be so kind. I finished college. I enrolled in graduate school.

Now, at thirty, my life is again reorganized. I have a medical past of sorts (ten years of negative checkups), which means I also have a prognosis—a favorable one. My hospital exams are now annual, although too many years of fearfulness still prevent me from making long-range plans. I have many close friends to whom I privately talk about cancer in a language neither furtive nor in-your-face confrontational, although I have learned that simply being able now to narrate the story in the past tense allows other people their concerned interest. Narrating a present and ongoing crisis, outcome unknown, is dangerous in any form of discourse.

More importantly, I am no longer completely self-referential. I am not immersed in a constant state of pain, physical or psychic. Every urination is not a premonition of disease. I do lapse into fits of worry about all possible bad fortunes (a worldview I call the "why NOT me?" syndrome). In general, my concerns are now connected to larger social issues, and I feel part of an ongoing human history. Teacher, feminist, environmentalist—I have a public self informed by political understandings.

This awareness has come to include a social perspective on cancer itself, my most private and dehumanizing experience. I know as a woman that having cancer alters one's physical and sexual self and is thus a gendered experience which requires a feminist analysis. I know as a cancer patient that different treatment options are made available according to perceived socio-economic status and possession of health insurance. I know as a biologist that the agents which cause cancer are found in the workplace, the home, the community, the food chain, our common environment—and that these are political and economic spheres.

The question for me now is, with these perspectives and experiences, why am I not a cancer activist? Why have I been, up to now, so silent? I am a published writer with a Ph.D. in science, which gives me a certain authority in this world of designated experts. I have been publicly and politically active on many other fronts. And yet when it comes to cancer . . . it's hard to focus. Apparently I would throw myself into any other social cause before I would take on this disease. With one in three of us falling victim to cancer at some point in our lives, I am intellectually convinced of the importance of cancer advocacy work. But then the paralysis sets in.

Many of those afflicted by AIDS become AIDS activists, deconstructing myths about the disease, organizing demonstrations, exposing government indifference, and fighting for patients' rights, access to drugs, and funding for research. Why am I not a cancer activist?

The question is partially rhetorical. A few years ago, while still a graduate student, I signed up as a teaching assistant for a new class called Biology of Cancer. This action was to be my first step towards a larger commitment as both scientist and activist to make cancer visible as a social issue. It was far from an empowering experience. Almost immediately, I started "forgetting" to attend lectures. When I did, I found myself sitting in the back row in a dark auditorium, overcome with anxiety, watching slide after slide of different tumor formations go by. Grading the papers and exams was excruciating. During my office hours nearly every student, it seemed, needed to tell me about the diagnosis of a parent or grandparent. I felt unable to counsel them, thinking only how they were the same age I was at the time of my own diagnosis. I became paranoid about my health. All of the curriculum development I had agreed to do went undone. I struggled with depression the entire semester and found other political activities on campus to redirect my commitments.

At least two things are clear to me now. First, working to expose cancer's public dimensions is itself largely an individual experience. There are resource centers which provide information about symptoms and detections, and there are support groups aimed at helping the victim cope with private stresses, but there are few cancer resource centers or organizations directed at the level of prevention or access to health care or environmental risk, for example. (The Women's Cancer Resource Center in Berkeley, California is an exception.) Thus there is little solidarity for this work. With so many of us out there, I am guessing this lack of a political movement around cancer probably means that others have experienced a paralysis similar to my own.

And this is the second point: working to make cancer a *public* issue—at least for me so far—carries with it the risk of being plunged back into the *private* hell of being a cancer victim.* The trick must be to uncouple somehow the socially visible from the

* Other authors have argued against the popular term "cancer victims" on the grounds that it reduces people with cancer to one-dimensional stereotypes, passive and helpless. I believe the term highlights the fact that cancer, as a preventable disease, is a human rights issue. Laws exist to prevent and punish other forms of criminal victimization; legislation that prevents and punishes victimization by environmental poisoning could dramatically reduce the incidence of cancer.

privately visible. To accomplish this separation, I think we first have to understand what the privately visible experience of cancer is and why it is so painful. In understanding it, perhaps we can move beyond it, which is what I am struggling to do now.

The private experience of cancer, that which involuntarily reorganizes our lives, is characterized by alternating swings between complete self-immersion and the reprieves of denial. In the immersion stage, we are engaged in a battle as we accommodate new information about our bodies and our futures, respond physically to our treatments, and make critical decisions under tremendous stress. As Audre Lorde has pointed out, we bring our whole historical self to bear on this process, including the inscriptions of our particular race, gender, and class.[4]

One key part of this battle for women, which I seldom hear discussed, is commanding oneself to submit to bodily invasions. Feminism has taught us how to reclaim our bodies, to celebrate them, to respect their integrity. Suddenly, we are required to consent to mutilation and painful treatment at the hands of strangers. We are asked to think of our body parts as potentially expendable, unimportant, not connected to the "self." This injunction seems regressive, part of an older, exploitative perspective. As one woman told me, "I worked a lifetime learning to accept my breasts, to believe they were beautiful, and now I am told I should just accept having them cut off."

A cancer victim can feel as though she has consented to rape or torture. The image of my own humiliation was the bloody catheter tube that extended from between my legs for two weeks after surgery. I slept curled around it, holding on to the plastic tube. When the tube moved, it moved inside me too, until the whole apparatus felt like an extension of my pain. At least twice daily it became clogged with blood clots and required "irrigation," a procedure which meant lying spread-eagled on the bed while whoever was available on the ward pumped syringes of water up into my bladder.

In the reprieve phase—after surgery or between treatments, biopsies, or exams—we want to deny and forget all that. And why not? The private experience of cancer means not being in control. We regain control when we are not confronted with the disease every single moment, when we can re-enter our other lives—social, sexual, and professional—if only temporarily. Even Audre Lorde, at the vanguard in constructing a political discourse on cancer, has described her own resistance to talking publicly about cancer during a time when she herself was trying to delay making crucial decisions about a possible liver metastasis:

> At the poetry reading in Zurich this weekend, I found it so much easier to discuss racism than to talk about *The Cancer Journals*. Chemical plants between Zurich and Basel have been implicated in a definite rise in breast cancer in this region, and women wanted to discuss this. I talked as openly as I could, but it was really hard. Their questions presume a clarity I no longer have.[5]

It is this blurring of vision that cancer victims have to overcome in order to talk and act publicly and politically. For me, the counterweight to my fears of returning to the life of the bloody catheter is the conviction that with knowledge comes responsibility. Learning to be a cancer activist means learning to get beyond the silence of reprieve in order to challenge the social and economic structures that allow cancer to lay claim to a third of us.

In my mind, there are at least three main battles around which we should be organizing. The first is to provide a challenge to the dominant rhetoric about cancer's causes and effects. This task requires a thorough understanding of the cancer research and medical establishments, particularly the American Cancer Society (ACS) and its government sibling, the National Cancer Institute (NCI). Public education campaigns of cancer establishments such as the ACS and the NCI focus almost exclusively on individual habit (diet, smoking, sunbathing, and breast self-exams) when addressing cancer prevention. This analysis never acknowledges that personal habits are themselves social constructions. But more importantly, an emphasis on lifestyle issues obscures the role of environmental hazards that are beyond personal choice. Workplace exposures alone are estimated to cause between 4 percent and 20 percent of all cancers, and well-documented cancer clusters have been mapped in communities located near chemical factories, refineries, nuclear reactors, and pesticide-saturated farm fields.[6] These are not randomly selected communities; they are, more often than not, poor and non-white. Of the 140,000 toxic waste dumps that have been identified in the United States, for example, 60 percent are located in Black or Hispanic neighborhoods.[7]

Nearly all mass-burn trash incinerators are located in impoverished communities, including the world's largest in Detroit.

Even industry spokespeople acknowledge that the toxic ash produced by the Detroit incinerator will raise the cancer incidence rate in the surrounding communities. This fact is not under dispute. The state of Michigan now estimates that the number of additional people who will contract cancer due to the incinerator exceeds the number of people employed by the incinerator.[8] The incinerator's victims will not die nice deaths; they will be amputated, irradiated, and dosed with chemotherapy. But they will expire privately in hospitals and will be buried quietly. We will not know who they are. Photographs of their bodies will not appear in the newspapers. Even they themselves will not know who they are.

I have a fantasy of covering the steps of the American Cancer Society headquarters with their bodies under a banner that reads, "Say something about trash incinerators." But, of course, it is the rest of us, the still living cancer victims, who must learn to say something, who must find a way to make these preventable deaths visible. For cancer institutions in a profit economy, raising money for pure cancer "research" will always take priority over exposing dangerous corporate practices.[9] And, since no one wants to donate to a losing cause, raising this money requires an optimistic public relations campaign. The ACS and the NCI have a stake in the public perception that we are "winning the war" on cancer, that a cure is just around the corner. They do not have a stake in publicizing the fact that the cancer incidence among American children has increased by 22 percent since 1950.[10]

The cancer establishment's almost doctrinaire emphasis on the importance of early detection also functions to obscure the social context of cancer. Popular articles frequently conflate detection with prevention, leading to spurious statements such as "Early detection is the best prevention!" Obviously, detecting cancer, no matter how early, makes irrelevant the possibility of preventing cancer. Early detection may prevent an earlier death, but it is not a vaccine against developing the disease.

Furthermore, the social issues surrounding the practice of early detection are seldom addressed. As a science writer for the *Detroit Free Press* in 1986, I reported on a university study which found that Black women with breast cancer in Detroit had markedly lower survival rates than white women. This difference was attributed to lack of early detection in the Black community, which in turn was attributed to a lower socio-economic status. It turns out that many poor women, a disproportionate number of whom are Black, could not afford to pay for mammograms. I proposed that we run a story on cancer mortality and the availability of health care. My editor rejected the idea as not sufficiently "sciency" enough for the science page. Instead, we ran a long comparative story on new surgical techniques for treating breast cancer. The detail about Detroit's different Black and white survival rates was buried somewhere in the middle of the article. This approach seems to me typical of most mass media stories on cancer; they reproduce, consciously or not, the cancer establishment's representation of cancer and its priorities (advances in new technologies over improving access to health care).

Neither the media nor the cancer establishment has had much to say about the stigmatization of cancer victims. Stigmatization, the process by which cancer victims adopt the status of the untouchable, is a third battle which needs taking on—not only because such disparagement is a matter of basic human rights, but because the stigmas themselves push cancer out of the visible world and deeper into obliterating silence and isolation. Stigmas are created by dominant social attitudes, but they are also reinforced and institutionalized by certain social structures which need to be changed. Three women writers by whom I have been inspired have already begun to expose this process.

Journalist and patients' rights advocate Jory Graham—not a particularly political person—directed her attention at the level of patient dignity and did much to improve social attitudes before her death in 1984. Graham worked to change what she called "the social climate" in which people with cancer live and make their decisions. Working together with medical professionals, she drew up a kind of constitutional bill of rights for patients. These included the right to accurate information about diagnosis and prognosis; the right to know treatment options; and the right to be free of pain. Fueled by her own rage at being lied to by her first oncologist (he felt it unnecessary to tell her about a lymph node metastasis found during her mastectomy), Graham's intent was to prohibit deceit at the level of the doctor-patient relationship and allow the patient free access to whatever chemical pain relievers are needed. With these conditions satisfied, the patient is empowered to participate in deciding her own treatment options.[11]

This bill of rights might be expanded to include the right to tell one's story publicly. Dorothea Lynch, another journalist now dead of breast cancer, found that she could be prevented from collecting testimony from patients living in a cancer ward through the invocation of "the right to patient privacy." Even in cases where people volunteered to be photographed and interviewed, doctors and hospital administrators frequently prohibited Lynch from entering patients' rooms or disrupted the interviews and cut them short in the name of "the right to privacy." Lynch suspected these measures were designed to prevent her from talking to certain patients whom she knew held critical views of the hospital or their treatment protocol. This perversion of the concept of "privacy" and its codification as an arbitrary hospital rule, Lynch wrote, functioned to thwart any public understanding of cancer and relegated the disease to the realm of secretiveness.[12] The imposed silence created by privacy regulations also, of course, keeps cancer victims from talking to each other and developing common understandings about their condition.

Audre Lorde deals with the specific stigmas associated with breast cancer. According to her now well-known and controversial analysis, post-mastectomy women are kept silent and separated from each other through the socially sanctioned prosthesis.[13] With one- and no-breasted women publicly stigmatized as freakish, the pressure to be normal forces women either to wear external prostheses or to submit to breast reconstruction. This process is self-perpetuating as women come to be ashamed of their altered bodies and hide them behind lumps of wool, cotton, or silicone, effectively and literally rendering breast cancer publicly invisible, confined to the realm of the secretive and stigmatized. The ACS reinforces this process, says Lorde, through its Reach to Recovery Program. In the meantime, money and energy which could be directed at prevention is spent researching techniques of breast reconstruction. Instead of reconstructing breasts, Lorde advocates reconstructing the legend of the single-breasted Amazon warrior as an alternative female model of power and beauty. In 1989, I saw Lorde speak at the University of Michigan. She was one-breasted, and she was indeed a powerful and lovely figure.

Some women I have talked with find Lorde's Amazon glorification and anti-prosthesis militancy insufficiently sensitive to working women, who face discrimination in the workplace, and to economically dependent wives, who risk losing their marriages. Single-breastedness, they say, is the choice of privilege.

Cancer victims learning to be cancer activists need to bring debates such as this one to the feminist community for public discussion. Thus far, we have let Audre Lorde do too much of this by herself. Within the feminist community, salient issues relating to women's cancer experiences can be publicized, interpreted, written about, organized around, and acted upon. Ultimately, a social construction of cancer can be collectively created to serve as an alternative to the cancer establishment's representations. With lung and breast cancer now the leading killers of women, sustained political attention from the women's community is absolutely essential.

I have heard it argued that women with cancer have little in common other than their disease—unlike members of the gay community organized around AIDS—and that this lack of objective bonds prevents an effective political response. There is probably some truth in this observation, but we need to understand and explore it further. It seems to me now, all myths of universal sisterhood aside, that a number of other powerful ties besides the disease itself bind us. First, women are still by and large the primary caretakers of children. Women thus have an important stake in the alarming rise in the cancer incidence in children. Second, the experience of cancer is a profoundly gendered experience in that it requires a rethinking of the relationship between the body and the self and between the self and other people. Feminist psychology, literature, and theory have already illuminated much about these relationships and also have had much to say about the development of shame, silence, passivity, and helplessness in women. Having cancer reproduces these conditions. We need feminist scholarship to help us understand how this happens.

The issues surrounding mammography and breast self-examination need to be debated in the women's community. We hear again and again how 90 percent of breast cancers are still discovered by women themselves, yet less than one-third of us examine our breasts regularly. We read these reports and feel guilty. But we never hear about what might prevent women from conducting self-exams. Lack of education? Uncertainty of what we're looking for? Shame of our bodies? The incredible conflict in seeking something we most dread to find? Many women's breast clinics now offer educational exams in which women can learn how to feel simulated breast lumps in silicone models. However, these sessions can cost upwards of $80.

The whole political economy of nuclear medicine needs to be

explicated. This investigation would include not only the prohibi-
tive cost of mammograms to poor women, as mentioned above,
but also their effectiveness as a tool of early detection. A baseline
mammogram is now recommended for *every* woman between the
ages of thirty-five and forty, and every few years after that.[14] Such
advice represents millions and millions of mammograms every
year. With the transportation and disposal of nuclear waste (much
low-level nuclear waste comes from hospitals) becoming a growing threat to public health in poorer communities, what do such
recommendations mean for preventing and detecting cancer in
women?

Finally, women with cancer need to be honest and open about
the issues that divide us. Age is an obvious one. Intellectually, I
know that ageism is an insidious form of discrimination in our
society, particularly for women. Older women are treated as dis-
posable in the workplace, in the community, and even in the
home. Older women with cancer are thus three times made invisible. Nevertheless, a younger woman with cancer can feel resentment at what seems to be the hegemony of older women and their
specific concerns within cancer support groups and the debates
at large. We younger women with cancer look at older women
and see that—whatever their prognosis—they have homes, children, spouses, a past life as a healthy adult, and friends old
enough to understand disease and mortality. Dorothea Lynch, at
thirty-four, wrote that she was having cancer at a time when
everyone else her age was having babies. ("I had felt diseased,
a carrier among the pregnant women with their different-sized
stomachs."[15]) At the age of twenty, I felt that I was having cancer
when everyone else was having sex. (I still maintain that returning
to a college dormitory room after cancer surgery is just about the
most depressing journey on earth.) Young women's concerns about
their reproductive health are often trivialized. A twenty-five-year-
old with leukemia, for example, wanted information on how the
chemotherapy treatments might affect her ovaries. Her doctor
replied that most people with leukemia do not plan to have children.[16] I have received similar comments.

Moreover, treatment protocols themselves are often based on
the assumption that the patient is older. For example, one of the
official recommendations for bladder cancer patients is an annual
kidney and bladder X-ray. Such a procedure, of course, has completely different implications for a sixty-year-old man than for a

twenty-year-old pre-reproductive female.

It is easier to get involved with refugees in Central America than with homelessness in your own city, I have often heard remarked. And so it is. Demonstrators step over the bodies of their invisible compatriots on their way to the protest. For me, dealing with the social implications of cancer can feel like being forced to look at my own body lying in the street—or, more accurately, curled around a catheter tube in a hospital bed. Nevertheless, this morning I read in the *Chicago Tribune* about the death from lung cancer of a forty-one-year-old woman nuclear power plant worker, and I feel the anger again, the need to speak out publicly. The article is not about this woman's life in the nuclear industry; her occupation is only mentioned in an incidental way somewhere in the middle of the story (just as in my own story about the higher mortality rate of Black women). The story I'm reading is about how this woman was pregnant and refused treatment for her disease for the sake of the baby. Soon after the baby was born, she died. What a wonderful woman, her surviving husband said, along with everyone else at her funeral. Thus, I am left to believe she sacrificed herself for her child, not for the nuclear power plant (which happens to be located thirty miles from my hometown). This oblation is the model I am given by the newspaper for women with cancer.

My memory goes back to the other woman with the resolute look in her eyes, still alive, holding her sign up to the camera: "We all live downwind." This is the model I take.

NOTES

1. Lynch, Dorothea, and Eugene Richards, "Amazon," *Granta*, No. 16, Summer 1985, p. 33.
2. Swift, Richard, "From This Month's Editor," *The New Internationalist*, No. 198, August, 1989, p. 3.
3. Lorde, Audre, *The Cancer Journals*, Aunt Lute Books, San Francisco, 1980, p. 2.
4. Lorde, pp. 9-10.
5. Lorde, Audre, *A Burst of Light*, Firebrand Books, Ithaca, NY 1988, p. 60.
6. Swift, Richard, "Breaking the Grip of Cancer," *The New Internationalist*, No. 198, August, 1989, p. 4.
7. *Toxic Waste and Race in the United States*, Commission for Racial Justice, United Church of Christ, 105 Madison Avenue, New York, NY 10016, 1987.
8. *Detroit News*, April 19, 1990, Sec. A, p. 1, col. 2.
9. Swift, p. 4.
10. National Cancer Institute statistic in Harper's Index, *Harper's*, March, 1990, p. 19.

11. Graham, Jory, *In the Company of Others: Understanding the Human Needs of Cancer Patients*, Harcourt Brace Jovanovich, New York, 1982, pp. 27-88.

12. Lynch and Richards, pp. 48-52.

13. Lorde, *The Cancer Journals*, pp. 55-77.

14. Holleb, Arthur I., M.D., *The American Cancer Society Cancer Book*, Doubleday & Co., New York, 1986, p. 253.

15. Lynch.

16. Geller, Matthew, *Difficulty Swallowing: A Medical Chronicle*, Works Press, New York, 1981, unpaginated.

Statistics

SANDY POLISHUK

"**D**on't worry, they tell us,
"Eighty-five percent of them
Are benign."

■

We let them cut,
Poison,
And burn.

We have blood tests,
X-rays,
And scans.

We visualize,
Exercise,
Give up fat.

There are no guarantees.

■

We compulsively examine
The lonely breast,
And pay too close attention
To every ache and twinge.

We buy organic produce,
Drink only bottled water,
But they don't sell air.

We are in awe
Of the energy we find
To fight it.

Which battle should we choose,
  The one within our bodies
  Or the larger one
  Out there?

We know there is a connection,
  This did not drop from the sky.

■

We shudder when someone else
  Has a recurrence,
  And guiltily sigh,
  "Not I,
  This time."

They tell us
  The greatest danger is
  In the first two years.

We have stopped believing in statistics.

Cancer as Violence Against Women

ADELE FRIEDMAN

We are a gentle, angry people . . .
—Holly Near

We were women and men brought together by our shared outrage at the violence against women in my home town of Rochester, New York, and by the violence against women in Montreal, and in Central America. We sang for our lives as we wove colored ribbons on which we wrote the names of victims into a memorial wreath. As I stood there by the table of ribbons, pen in hand, the angry words broke through my composed serenity and wrote themselves: "Edith, you never had a chance."

Edith is my mother. She died from breast cancer. It took that memorial gathering, with its focus on the killing of women just because they were women, to force upon me the essential connection of those women to me and mine. I thought of the death from cancer of my mother, of my own recent encounter with the disease, of the growing threat to the lives of my sister, my two daughters, and my friends. Breast cancer is an unchecked epidemic in this country.

The annual number of women newly diagnosed with breast cancer in 1989 alone is significantly greater than the total number of AIDS deaths since they were first recorded in 1980, and breast cancer death rates are increasing.[1], [2] The mortality statistics from breast cancer have risen for women born into each succeeding decade of this century. Women born in the 1930s, like me, have a higher rate of breast cancer than women born in the 1920s.[3] And this steady swell continues despite the proclaimed improved odds for survival attributed to chemotherapy.[4]

One specialist with a national reputation in breast cancer treatment stated, "With the rising incidence of breast cancer, no matter how well you treat it, the death rate is going to go up."[5] And if you treat breast cancer ineptly or don't treat it at all, the death rate rises more steeply.

Why is this anguish allowed to continue? Just as the women we honored that night had been slain because women's lives—and our deaths—are of little value in the eyes of so many men, we, too, are victims of a national agenda established by leaders with a woefully inadequate regard for the ravages of a disease which afflicts women almost exclusively. The leaders who define our priorities and prepare our budgets do not consider that the killing of 43,000 women in one year (1988) constitutes a national crisis. On the contrary; in 1986 our government diverted $105 million from saving lives to taking lives as they cut funds for the National Cancer Institute by as much as the funds secretly diverted to the Contras.[6]

Women, who are the present and potential victims of this particular violence of neglect and indifference, seem to acquiesce in our national disregard for women's lives. Too often, we are docile accomplices in our fates. Despite the many thousands of us who develop breast cancer every year, the one in nine American women who constitute those annual figures does so within a cultural context which dictates that cancer is "an unavoidable misfortune which we as isolated individuals must accept."[7]

Certainly I count myself as having been among the ranks of women who accepted breast cancer as foreordained for me. My heritage from my mother, which gave me some of my most valued gifts and strengths, also gave me—I thought—breast cancer. If I could accept and relish the praiseworthy qualities I inherited from her, I felt I was not free to refuse the cancer. I had to pay the price. Besides my mother's cancer, I had other "risk factors," too, and I valued them as I valued my heritage from my mother: I had just turned fifty, I am Jewish, and I had lived most of my life in Northeastern cities.[8]

On the other hand, I had done all the right things when I had any real choices to make, and it wasn't until later that I learned my lifestyle choices were extolled as excellent cancer preventatives. I'd been a vegetarian with a low-fat, high-fiber diet for many years. I had given birth to three children in my late twenties, and I had breast-fed them. When things got tough, rather than smoke or drink I would write and play slow Brahms. I did not take birth control pills, and I had refused estrogen replacement therapy. Yet, when I received my cancer diagnosis, I wasn't surprised that heredity and environment had won out over clean living.

During a reunion with an epidemiologist friend a year following my surgery, I recited to her my litany of risk factors and preventive measures. She shook my equanimity by stating that the single greatest risk factor was chance. Since breast cancer is almost exclusively a disease of women, I understood her declaration to mean that my single greatest risk factor for contracting one of the three largest cancer-killers was having been born a woman. [9]

In the manner dictated by my culture, I was sweetly reasonable when I was confronted with the necessity for a bilateral mastectomy. Certainly it is true that the reserves of calm and optimism on which I drew were essential to my survival from the physical and psychological ordeal I underwent: first the sentence of the disease itself and then the surgery and chemotherapy that I hoped would eradicate it. "There is no problem without a gift for you in its hands," reads the quote from J. S. Bach on my reconstructive surgeon-violinist's wall. I agree. My experience with cancer did bring me gifts. I gained freedom from many of the expectations placed on me by other people because I could no longer continue on as I had. I gained freedom to express myself without the usual reservations about what I said and to whom. I was well rewarded for my openness about my condition and its treatment from other survivors and from my friends and family. I received an outpouring of care and affection from people who shared with me the liberation which comes from a confrontation with mortality.

There is some evidence that a supportive community plays an important role in the success of treatment for disease. The impact of emotional support is not only psychological, but appears to have biological implications as well. A woman's perception of strong social support appears to be the best predictor of the effectiveness of her body's natural killer cells in the attack against her cancer. [10] I was lucky; I had love and support. As I regained my health and strength, I thought I should share my understanding of this aspect of recovery with others by writing about it.

But the words would not come. As I continued to read and think about the experience of breast cancer, there were too many facts which did not fit neatly into the sunny picture I was coloring. I had wanted my emphasis to be on how to take control of one's life through open communication and establishing vital connections to other people. But how could I integrate into this model the statistics which show that the breast cancer epidemic is clearly out of control? How could I account for the refusal of the medical/

nutritional establishment to acknowledge the mounting evidence of the role of a low-fat diet in the prevention of breast cancer?[11] How could I explain the attempts by plastic and reconstructive surgeons and the manufacturers of silicone implants used in breast reconstruction to suppress experimental data, resist regulation, and squelch discussion about the possible risks involved?[12,13] What of the Federal Drug Administration's decision to risk feeding hormones to breast cancers in their earliest, non-palpable stage through lifting the recommended upper age limit for oral contraceptives?[14] And, when I looked honestly at my own experience, how could I ignore the implications of the way in which my general surgeon nearly deprived me of any decision-making power at the very onset of the treatment process?

When my surgeon discussed my options with me at our final meeting before my scheduled admission to the hospital, he failed to distinguish between breast preservation (through lumpectomy followed by radiation) and reconstruction. I thought that the size and location of the tumor identified through the needle biopsy had ruled out preservation as an option for me. The surgeon didn't describe exactly what the physical results of the mastectomy would be, and he never mentioned reconstruction as a possibility. I made what I thought was a logical assumption: if there was not going to be enough remaining of my breast to preserve, then there wouldn't be enough tissue left for reconstruction either. I didn't know enough to ask more questions about reconstruction, and the surgeon—who assuredly did—didn't bother to tell me.

By accident, I learned that reconstruction was, in fact, a possibility for me, and that the process could be started during the mastectomy operation to avoid another major surgery. The nurse practitioner who was preparing me for admission to the hospital had had a mastectomy and breast reconstruction ten years before, and when she discovered that I had never been informed or consulted about reconstruction, she immediately got my surgeon on the telephone. He apologized for having forgotten to mention reconstruction; like too many surgeons—particularly with middle-aged women—he just assumed that I wasn't interested.[15] He then scratched the scheduled surgery and the hospital admission and arranged for me to see a reconstructive surgeon. My mastectomy was rescheduled, this time with both surgeons attending.

While testicular and penile implants have always been covered by Massachusetts Blue Cross/Blue Shield, women had to fight to secure coverage for post-mastectomy reconstruction to be class-ified as "rehabilitation" rather than as a not-covered elective cosmetic surgery.[16] And were I a man with cancer of the prostate, for instance, I think it is unlikely that my surgeon would have forgotten to assure that I had access to information about the new surgical techniques which minimize or eliminate the risk of impo-tence as a result of the therapeutic operation.

I felt as though I had been pulled back from a precipice at the last possible moment before being pushed over the edge—into a decision based on inadequate information which would set a course I did not choose to follow. I was grateful to the admitting nurse practitioner for having returned to me a measure of control over my body and my treatment. But I remained seriously troubled by what my personal experience meant for other women. Luck had played such a large part in making me aware of my options; other women might not be so lucky.

I do have the power to help a few women who have been diagnosed with breast cancer. I can help them figure out what questions to ask their physicians before deciding on a course of treatment. The medical profession will not look so kindly on this early intervention in their cherished "doctor-patient relationship" as they do on the mainstream visits of Reach to Recovery volun-teers after surgery. Doctors communicate to their patients an urgency about surgery unsupported by what we know of the years it takes a tumor to grow. I hope that by working through local support groups I can both legitimatize my efforts to counsel women before surgery and minimize the isolation which keeps women with cancer feeling weak and ineffectual.

But reducing the numbers of women who receive that unwel-come diagnosis in the first place will take work to influence policy-making at the national level. Although breast cancer repre-sents 14 percent of all cancers and 28 percent of the cancer in women in the United States, it receives just 4 percent of the research dollars.[17] Throwing more money at the problem is not enough, however. Rather, we need a basic shift in the way we approach it. Instead of continuing the costly search for the magic bullet, a search which has dominated the national "war on cancer," we should urge that research dollars be reapportioned to address the reality of our current situation. "Because cures for most cancers are not likely in the near future, focusing so much money and energy on treatment research may be actually robbing us of the motivation and resources to try to prevent cancer."[18]

. We do not use the knowledge we already possess about preventing breast cancer and diminishing its effects. For instance, the certification of mammography facilities is now voluntary, and the American College of Radiology has so far certified fewer than a quarter of the facilities in this country.[19] Yet radiation in excess of the one rem recommended maximum* poses a particular hazard, since "except for the developing fetus, the female breast is the most radiosensitive of all human tissues."[20] Despite this danger, no federal laws regulate the use of diagnostic equipment or the qualifications of operators.

We need the full and accurate dissemination of the considerable body of scientific evidence concerning the fat/cancer connection in preventing breast cancer and the recurrence of lesions elsewhere in the body.[21] As Susan Rennie has documented, this information has not been made public because of the influence of special interest groups (nutritionists and physicians with ties to the meat and dairy lobbies), and the conservative leadership of the American Cancer Society and the National Cancer Institute.[22] The latter organization is still doing a "feasibility study" to determine whether women at high risk for breast cancer are in fact capable of acting in their own interest by following a regime with a dietary fat level low enough to make a difference in breast cancer prevention: twenty percent or less of total caloric intake, half the standard American level. They report "good compliance."[23]

From my own hard-fought battle with cancer, I have learned that turning inward to tap deep sources of spiritual strength and drawing comfort from those closest to us allow us to attain a level of serenity and hope which promotes healing. When the enemy has retreated, however, a different tactic is needed, for the attitudes and strategies which helped one contend with the personal challenge posed by a diagnosis of cancer can blur one's perception of the underlying social problem. The objectives now change from coping with assault to actively securing the fortress against future attacks. This transformation requires turning those horrifying statistics of our vulnerability into a source of strength in numbers.

* *Editor's Note:* By comparison, a typical chest X-ray is about .03 rem—much, much lower than the typical mammogram, even under the best of circumstances. The real problem is that there are no universally employed standards for mammographic equipment and technicians. Dr. Edward Hendricks said on the NBC Nightly News (June 22, 1990), "In roughly fifty percent of the places, mammography sites, there's not adequate quality assurance going on."

Such a reversal will not be easy for us. We women tend to be gentle. But in the face of injustice, we can also be an angry people. That is why it is necessary for us to understand that the current epidemic of breast cancer is one form of institutionalized violence against women.

NOTES

1. Centers for Disease Control, HIV Information Line, March 1, 1990.

2. American Cancer Society, *Cancer Facts and Figures—1989*, p. 8.

3. Hahn, Robert A., M.D., "Deaths from Breast Cancer Among Women—United States, 1986," Centers for Disease Control: *Morbidity and Mortality Weekly Report* 38:33, August 25, 1989, pp. 565-569.

4. "Studies Cite Benefits of Chemotherapy in Early Breast Cancer," *New York Times*, February 23, 1989.

5. "Breast cancer death rate is up and highest in Northern states," *Times-Union*, Rochester, New York, August 25, 1989.

6. Lorde, Audre, *A Burst of Light*, Firebrand Books, Ithaca, New York, 1989, p. 133.

7. Brady, Judith, call for manuscripts, "Anthology on Women and Cancer," 1989.

8. Kushner, Rose, *Alternatives: New Developments in the War on Breast Cancer*, Warner Books, New York, 1987, p. 104.

9. Young, Wende Logan, M.D., on "The Talk Show," (WXXI-AM, Rochester, New York, April 11, 1989): "The biggest risk factor is simply that you are an aging woman."

10. Finkelstein, Harry, "Psychosocial Predictors of Breast Cancer Outcome," *COPE*, November, 1988.

11. Rennie, Susan, "Breast Cancer Prevention: A Controversial New Diet Program," *Ms.*, April, 1987, pp. 40-88.

12. Blakeslee, Sandra, "Breast Implant Surgery: More Facts Are Sought in the Battle Over Safety," *New York Times*, December 18, 1989.

13. Zones, Jane Sprague, "The Dangers of Breast Augmentation," *The Network News*, National Women's Health Network, July/August, 1989, pp. 1-8.

14. Fugh-Berman, Adriane, M.D., "Should Women Over Forty Take the Pill?" *The Network News*, p. 4.

15. "Advances in Breast Reconstruction Ease the Trauma of Cancer Surgery," *New York Times*, January 21, 1988.

16. Kushner, p. 388.

17. Porcino, Jane, Ph.D., *Growing Older, Getting Better: A Handbook for Women in the Second Half of Life*, Addison-Wesley, Reading, Massachuusetts, 1983, p. 162.

18. Bailar III, John C., and Elaine M.Smith, "Progress Against Cancer," *The New England Journal of Medicine*, May 8, 1986, pp. 1226-1232.

19. Monroe, Linda Roach, "A new focus on breast cancer: groups step up efforts for standards in mammography," reprinted from the *Los Angeles Times* in the *Times-Union*, Rochester, New York, December 5, 1989.

20. Kushner, pp. 388-389.

21. "Diet may count even after breast cancer develops," *Tufts University Diet & Nutrition Letter* 7:11, January, 1990, p. 1.

22. Rennie.

23. National Cancer Institute—FY 1988 Budget (excerpt from the Congressional Justification), March 1987, p. 8.

Smile, You've Got Breast Cancer!

SHARON BATT

A t the fifth annual AIDS conference in Montreal, in June of 1989, AIDS activists interrupted sessions with pointed questions, booed boastful scientists and politicians, demanded faster progress, and called for a moment of silence in memory of the dead.

It was an unprecedented show of patient power.

More often, the response to a frightening diagnosis is to keep a low profile. Prejudices about the life-threatening illness can put one's job at risk, snap even strong social ties, and throw into jeopardy a whole range of other benefits which the healthy take for granted. Silence offers a safer course, but the silent are also powerless. AIDS activists have recognized this social reality; they succinctly state the case for speaking out with a button proclaiming, "Silence = Death."

When I heard my diagnosis of breast cancer in 1988, I told only a few close friends whose support I needed to carry me through the initial chaos. The morning I had the lump removed from my breast, I called my boss from the hospital lobby and said that I had to have "a few medical tests." By that noon I knew the chickpea-sized mass removed from my breast was malignant, but the next day I was back at my desk as if nothing had happened. During the ensuing weeks a tornado of cancer thoughts whirled though my head. But whenever that ubiquitous question, "How are you?" came my way, I felt my face form into a smile and I heard my voice chirp brightly, "I'm fine—I'm just fine!"

Two kinds of pressure combined to end my silence. The schizophrenia became unbearable. As I was play-acting my old self— the me who dashed out of the office at noon to go skiing, the forty-three-year-old who was often mistaken for thirty, the chronically well person who hadn't spent a night at a hospital since having an appendectomy at age eleven—my new self, me with cancer, was struggling for definition. Making sense of my altered self would be hard under the best of circumstances; wrapped in an ever-thickening cocoon of lies, it was impossible.

Another pressure to break the silence mounted as my frantic reading taught me more about breast cancer. I realized how abysmally ignorant I had been about this common killer of women. Of course I had known about breast self-examination for about as long as I had had breasts, and I knew that finding a lump was a menacing sign. The phrase "the mutilation of mastectomy" stuck in my mind as the gruesome, but ultimately bearable, sequel to finding a malignant lump—though I was dimly aware that even this horrific prospect was no longer inevitable.

What had not really crossed my mind, however, was that women—women of my age, especially—died of this disease. I had an aunt who died of breast cancer, but she was in her sixties. A few days after my lumpectomy I read a university thesis about breast cancer (the library had only one real book on the subject, and it was thirteen years old). The author of the thesis, freed from the constraint of having to woo readers, did not fool around with euphemisms. In clinical detail she described "the inevitable trajectory" to death of 50 percent of the women in her study. When those words finally cracked the wall around my resisting consciousness, the book flew out of my hands across the room. Nauseous, I reeled about my apartment in a daze for the rest of the day. Finally I understood that I might die, in my forties, of cancer.

In the months that followed my diagnosis, I began to open up to friends and even acquaintances, and I learned that most of these people knew no more about breast cancer than I had. "YOU have cancer? But you look fine!" More than one friend revealed basic confusions about chemotherapy and radiotherapy. "What's chemotherapy? Is that where they zap you with a big machine?" In low voices people asked me, "Did they get it all out?" They seemed amazed as I explained the significance of my one positive lymph node, and why it was that I had no way of knowing whether the chemotherapy was killing the cells circulating in my body. No one was so bold as to ask me if my breast was gone. Instead they delicately groped, "Did you have . . . aahh . . . surgery?" If I volunteered that I had, but that the scar was already nearly invisible, I was met with a gaze of polite skepticism. Breast cancer in most people's heads is synonymous with a Frankenstein-like slash across the torso.

The more I talked to people about breast cancer, the more impatient I became with their wide-eyed wonder about the disease. After all, this was not some rare condition that I had picked up on a foreign holiday. In North America, breast cancer is the main killer of women aged forty to fifty-five. Then why do so many people know so little about it?

Superficially, those of us with the disease have come a long way since the mid-1970s, when two prominent political wives, Betty Ford and Happy Rockefeller, announced to the world that they had undergone mastectomies. Other high-profile women have since come out of the breast cancer closet, making it easier for all women to follow. Even so, most women would rather suffer the "disgrace" of cancer and breastlessness privately. Few of us would fight to be heard at a cancer conference.

In the 1980s, the prescribed attitude for women with breast cancer was stoic optimism. That requisite cheerfulness is a small, sideways step from silence.

Breast cancer remains one of the three big cancer killers in North America. For women it has long been the number one cancer killer, ahead of lung and colon cancer. Lung cancer deaths, which are rising dramatically, now compete for first place.[1] The mortality rate for breast cancer has remained stable in the past fifty years at between 33 and 50 percent (depending on how the statistics are calculated), while the incidence seems to be increasing.[2] The average age of breast cancer onset is dropping, with more and more women under thirty being diagnosed.[3]

Although considered one of the more survivable cancers,[4] the sheer number of deaths annually is staggering because so many women—one in nine—get the disease. The most recent Canadian figures show that 4,350 women and thirty-one men died of breast cancer in 1987.[5] Compare these statistics to the 417 deaths from AIDS in Canada in the same year.[6]

Given these numbers, women with breast cancer might be expected to wield even more political clout than people with AIDS. It simply hasn't been so. We have not mobilized to make our illness a political issue. In Canada, women have not spoken as openly about breast cancer as American women have since the Ford and Rockefeller declarations. And no one, on either side of the border, has organized anything like a project to stitch the names of breast cancer victims into a quilt for posterity as the AIDS community has done for its dead.

Instead, the current vogue is to be hopeful, even chipper, about breast cancer. Much fanfare is made, for instance, of research demonstrating that mastectomies are unnecessary in many early-diagnosed cases. In practice, however, many surgeons routinely lop off the entire breast because that is the technique they learned in medical school. And while treatment options have expanded beyond simple surgery (radiation, chemotherapy and hormonal treatments have joined surgery in the medical establishment's arsenal), the odds of surviving breast cancer have scarcely improved in fifty years.[7,8]

Effects of the new treatments are still open to debate; most are still in the testing stage. Nevertheless—as the numbers stricken continue to rise—women are encouraged to be optimistic about their chances, to press bravely ahead with their lives as if death were out of the question, and to choose among available treatments as if out shopping for a new dress.

An American television broadcast, "Destined to Live," aired in June of 1989, illustrates this upbeat perspective. The program presented several dozen women and one man talking about their experiences with the disease. They spoke movingly about their initial terror at the moment of diagnosis, but most maintained they had conquered their fear of cancer. Pithy, bright messages dotted the testimonials. "When life kicks you, let it kick you forward," advised a woman who had survived a year and two months. "I laughed at it and I beat it, that's all," said the man, who is still alive eleven years after his diagnosis. "With breast cancer especially, patients make the difference, not the physicians," said a two-year survivor, feminist Gloria Steinem.

Everyone felt—and looked—great. They had chosen the treatments that were "right" for them. Husbands were supportive, friends were loving, careers flourished as never before. Doctors inspired total faith. One young woman was shown yachting with her oncologist. Several other women had given birth to healthy children since their diagnoses. A syrupy theme song gushed, "Brand new dreams, I'm filled with brand new dreams. They're more than dreams; they're coming true!"

Courage is all very well; anyone facing cancer certainly needs fortitude. But the picture presented by the television program was at best one-sided. Patients who felt sick were not heard from. Those who died were neither mentioned nor mourned. Completely missing from the broadcast was any hint that the public should be concerned about breast cancer. The notion of "treatment choice" was absurdly simplified. The message was: shop for Doctor Right, and an effective treatment is yours. The seductive concept that patient optimism cures cancer—which is still very much theory, not fact—bathed the personal stories in a rosy glow.

The price of this Pollyanna stance is political impotence. Media attention to breast cancer bears little relation to reality. Support services for women with cancer remain meager.

Women diagnosed with breast cancer can learn a lot from the AIDS activists. We can push for better educational programs, for more research into causes and treatments, for more information on how—and how much—money is spent. Women with breast cancer can choose to be openly critical of the current emphasis on expensive cosmetic devices: wigs to hide hair loss during chemotherapy, breast implants of questionable safety, and over-priced silicone bra-stuffers (top-of-the-line models now feature nipples, for that perky look). It's tempting to participate in the subterfuge of looking near-perfect even when your life is at risk, but the costs go far beyond the millions of dollars drained from our collective bank accounts. These tricks to keep surgery and baldness secret make us invisible to each other and to society at large. They contribute to the lie that breast cancer is a piffling disease which can easily be relegated to one's past. They encourage silence rather than protest.

As American writer Audre Lorde put it, "What would happen if an army of one-breasted women descended upon Congress and demanded that the use of carcinogenic fat-stored hormones in beef-feed be outlawed?"[9] Breast cancer patients can't afford to be complacent. Let's drop the pose that we're one happy, beautiful bunch of survivors.

NOTES

1. Age-standardized mortality rates for Canadian women, as reported in *Canadian Cancer Statistics 1989*, p. 27, show breast cancer as the highest (with a rate per 100,000 population fluctuating between 23 and 25 throughout the period of 1970 to 1987), while lung cancer rises from about 6 per 100,000 in 1970 to 19 per 100,000 in 1987). At a June, 1989 symposium on cancer in Saskatoon, Dr. William Evans, Director of the Regional Cancer Centre in Ottawa, stated that lung cancer had surpassed breast cancer as the number one killer of women (reported in the Montreal Gazette, July 3, 1989, p. C7).

2. *Canadian Cancer Statistics 1989*, National Cancer Institute of Canada, Toronto, Canada, 1989, p. 26. The incidence of breast cancer (women only) was at 62 per 100,000 in 1970 and 71 per 100,000 in 1984.

3. Kushner, Rose, *Alternatives*, Warner Books, New York, 1984, p. 66.

4. *Canadian Cancer Statistics 1989*, p. 33. This publication lists five-year survival rates in Canada for breast cancer at 74 percent, while the survival rate for colon cancer is 51 percent and for lung cancer, 15 percent.

5. *Canadian Cancer Statistics 1989*, p. 19.

6. Telephone conversation with Health and Welfare Canada.

7. Boston Women's Health Collective, *Our Bodies, Ourselves*, Simon & Shuster, Inc., New York, 1984, p. 531.

8. Kushner, p. 65.

9. Lorde, Audre, *The Cancer Journals*, Aunt Lute Books, San Francisco, 1980, p. 16.

II. Not Even as Safe as Mother's Milk: The Environmental Connection

All I Know

SANDY POLISHUK

They tell us it's an acceptable risk,
Only three per million.

All I know is
I have cancer.

Last month I heard about
Three more friends,
And one so far this month.

My parents didn't get cancer,
Nor their friends,
At our age.

I am tired of band-aids,
Of focus on cures.
I want the causes removed,
Prevention at the source.

I want health above profits,
I want regulation over growth.
I want priorities for the long haul.

I want my grandson to grow up
And walk in a rain forest.
I want birds to lay eggs
That hatch.

All I know is
Acceptable risk
Is unacceptable thinking.
Throw the bums out.

Ostriches of the World, Unite!

NANCY BRUNING

"That's why I don't read the newspapers—it's too depressing. I'd go out and start shooting people."

That's my husband, Michael, speaking. I had just been reading out loud about the latest environmental atrocity. It doesn't matter which atrocity; they all come down to the same thing: greed, stupidity, and apathy taking their toll on "innocent" bystanders.

But we are rapidly losing our innocence. Anyone with eyes and ears knows that our environment is being poisoned and degraded at breakneck speed while big business and big government are still mouthing the same lame excuses: "That's progress," or "We're creating much-needed jobs," or "Whoops—we didn't know." Michael is right. It *is* depressing. It *does* make you want to shoot people—anyone, just so you don't feel so helpless, so victimized.

Depressing as all that is, I found it even more depressing and enraging to be diagnosed with cancer, especially breast cancer at the age of thirty-one. There was no breast cancer in my family, and I was a healthy, active, robust young woman. What is going on here?

Suddenly I was hearing, "You need a mastectomy": off with your breast! "You need chemotherapy": out with your hair, away with your get-up-and-go; what's a little constant nausea for nine months?

I lost my innocence nine years ago when I lost my health and began to make connections. The connection between my disease and breathing polluted air, eating a high-fat diet rich in antibiotic- and hormone-laden meat, smoking cigarettes to be cool and lose weight, and taking birth control pills which the medical profession assured me were safe; the connection between the need to sell a "product" at all costs and the production of the terrifying, life-threatening illness within me. Ohmigod—you mean there is a connection between the health of the earth and the health of the creatures (like me) living on it?

It's sad, but true, that most of us have to be struck directly and dramatically in order to make connections or begin to do something about the correlations we have already understood. But even after drastic treatment or a poor prognosis, so many victims of cancer go about their business, trying to get back to living life as usual, life as it was before cancer. I do not understand that effort to deny our own experiences; surely we should fight back when punched in the gut, no?

I suppose it's somewhat understandable if the still healthy remain unmoved by what is happening around them. But it's important to wake up to the fact that we are all affected indirectly by the impact of an increasingly polluted earth, and there is a growing probability that we or our loved ones will be the next statistic. As our environment becomes overburdened with pollution, so do our bodies. The earth—and its inhabitants—can handle only so much until the breaking point is reached.

Yes, Michael, shooting people may be tempting, but it isn't the answer. Neither is avoiding newspapers and sticking your head in the sand, ostrich-fashion. The desire to evade reality is almost understandable on the part of the average healthy person, but I do not see how a person with cancer can go back to the same old life, the same old attitudes, the same way of seeing the world. Perhaps getting back to normal is better than shooting people, but in a way it's the same thing. Different means, same result: people suffer and die.

Our planet is on the verge of losing the ability to clean and regenerate itself; pollution is everywhere. DDT has been found as far away as in the penguins of Antarctica.[1] We aren't penguins, but we are all guinea pigs involuntarily playing our parts in the largest and most dangerous enterprises ever devised. We may not realize the harm in our actions, but what we do has consequences whether we know it or not. For instance, burning fossil fuel (that is, driving a car) contributes to the greenhouse effect which probably exacerbated 1988's summer drought,[2] which in turn led to the growth of the potent carcinogen aflatoxin in corn,[3] and that corn found its way into the breakfast cereal and milk on our kitchen tables.

What happens on a large scale touches us locally. Disasters like the greenhouse effect may seem insurmountable, overwhelming in their complexity, magnitude, and number. The difficulty is that when people roll over and play dead, they run the very real risk that they may end up dead for real. Given those odds, any action, no matter how small, is better than nothing. And today we have many options and outlets for positive action. There's no longer any excuse for choosing passivity and silence. What's more, a healthier environment improves our lives by helping us reconnect with the earth "in ways that bring us joy as well as preserve natural resources."[4]

The important fact to remember is this: to make a difference, we need to think globally and act locally. We *can* take measures to protect ourselves from the pollution which already exists, and we *can* act to reduce the formation of pollution in the future. That sounds like a tall order, but as I began to understand that connection between my cancer and the world in which I live, I found ways to make changes. When I shop for food, I usually buy organic produce. If my grocer doesn't stock it, I ask him to. When an environmental group such as Greenpeace or the Natural Resources Defense Council sends me material in the mail, I don't throw it away; I read it, educate myself, and send a contribution. I'm gradually replacing toxic household products with safer ones. I investigated the recycling programs where I live and recycle newspapers and glass. I know my area has problems with contaminants in the water, so I bought a good filter, and I also let my government representatives know that I want my water cleaned up at the source. I know my local environmental groups, and I keep my eyes and ears open for local pollution infractions.

I've invested my meager savings in Working Assets, one of the growing number of socially conscious money markets. There are even checking accounts and credit cards that will donate a specific amount to environmental organizations with every check or purchase. I refer to the booklet *Shopping for a Better World*[5] so I can keep up with companies that have good track records of environmentally sound practices and avoid buying from companies with poor records. I also write to those company presidents to say why I refuse to buy their products. In election years, I make it my business to find out where the candidates stand. I tell my representatives my concerns about environmental pollution, and I tell them that it's worth whatever it will cost to control it. I support them when they stand up for all of our rights to a cleaner, safer world, and I let them know that I will fight against their election if they do not take strong positions against poisoning the earth.

I don't mean to imply that we can't have any fun. The more I learn, the more obvious it is that a little creativity and imagination can go a long way in cleaning up the environment. For example, a friend of mine recently gave herself a birthday party at which the preferred "gift" to her was a donation to an environmental group. One of my neighborhood groups recently organized a local tree-planting event to beautify the streets and help clean the air. Nature walks combined with clean-up brigades are fun and environmentally "profitable" too, as is inviting an environmentalist to speak to a local social group. I ride my bike or walk whenever possible because I really enjoy these activities. There are almost always less-polluting solutions available—witness the switch to ink made from soybeans instead of newspaper ink containing dangerous heavy metals.

Spreading the word about the potential dangers in environmental pollution is important. Since it is easier to learn than to unlearn, it is crucial that we help children see the connections and become involved. Children have the most to lose by inheriting a polluted future. I want to do what I can to encourage the children in my life to think about the consequences of their actions, and to consider jobs and careers in fields that are nonpolluting or that help reduce pollution. Schools and activity groups can plan educational and activist lessons and trips (visiting an eye-opening dump or landfill, for instance). Children need to know that you are never too small or too young to make a difference. College students have participated in a week-long demonstration to promote concern for the environment;[6] a fifteen-year-old instigated a move to stop the use of polystyrene trays in the school cafeteria.[7]

Fortunately, many diverse present and future dangers from pollution can be dealt with in broad strokes. Eating less meat reduces the pesticide, hormone, and antibiotic residues in our bodies and reduces fat intake; it lowers fossil fuel consumption, spares grain for use as human food rather than animal fodder, and reduces the deforestation of Central America to create new cattle ranches. Riding a bike or walking supports immune functions by giving us an emotional life and reducing fat in our bodies; it saves energy and pollutes less, too. Choosing public transportation over driving our own cars reduces the poisons we breathe which come from burning gasoline.

I've already been hit with cancer, as have millions of other people. I am one of the lucky ones—I'm still here, still fighting. As more and more people take a stand against pollution and the polluters, our children will have a greater chance of escaping the game of cancer roulette. I know my small contributions alone won't save the world, but maybe I can help save a part of it. Like pebbles in a pond, our actions make a ripple effect which touches other people and other events. Just as pollutants accumulate in our bodies to cause harm, so many people and small actions can add up to effect big changes.

NOTES

1. Davidson, Keay, "Journey to the End of the Earth," *San Francisco Examiner*, Jan. 8, 1989, p. A-10.
2. Begley, Sharon, "The Endless Summer?" *Newsweek*, July 11, 1989, p. 18.
3. Robbins, William, "Drought Sets Off Alarms on U.S. Response to Enemy of Corn," *New York Times*, March 2, 1989.
4. "How the Environmental Crisis Can Improve Our Lives," *Utne Reader*, Nov./Dec. 1989, p. 69.
5. Published by the Council on Economic Priorities, 30 Irving Place, New York, NY 10003.
6. "Fostering Concern for the Environment," *New York Times*, Oct. 23, 1989, p. B6.
7. James, George, "A Revolutionary Idea: Schools' Plastics Ban," *New York Times*, April 28, 1989, p. A16.

The Harvest of Poison

REINA DIAZ

We are always told in this country that it is our fault if we should get cancer. Everywhere you look there are articles in popular magazines telling you that if you eat carrots, don't drink coffee, and don't smoke you won't get cancer.

Well, I don't like to eat carrots. I do drink coffee, and I do smoke. I was also diagnosed as having cancer of the stomach only a few years ago. I guess I am supposed to believe it's my fault that I got that cancer.

So far as any of us knows, there was never any cancer in my family on either my mother's or my father's side. It was a big shock to me and my family when two-thirds of my stomach had to be removed. And when you consider that out of thirteen children, two of us—one of my brothers and myself—had stomach cancer and one sister had ovarian cancer, the shock is supplanted by growing doubts and some serious concern for what is going on here.

When I asked the surgeon who removed the major portion of my stomach how long he thought that cancer had been growing in me, he told me that he guessed about two years. Two years? I don't think so. No one knows exactly where my cancer came from, but I think that cancer had been lying in wait for a long time before it became a detectable mass. Just as I think that part of the reason for my recovery from such a serious cancer lies in the powerful love and support which I got from my family, so I also think the cause of that cancer can be found in the conditions under which I had to live most of my life—the same conditions under which most farmworkers still live.

At the time my cancer was finally diagnosed, I had not been a farmworker for many years. I have no idea whether or not the years spent in the fields or the cannery had anything to do with my cancer, though I cannot help but wonder. Long and concentrated exposure to toxic substances surely has had some effect on my body's ability to fight off disease.

My history has been one of working in the dirt and of eating dirt, a history of poverty and pesticides. I was one of thirteen children. My parents were both born in Mexico, but they met and married in the United States, and then traveled with my father's family in caravans all throughout the Southwest, working in the fields. They came into California through Indio and settled in Upland, outside Los Angeles, where I was born. When I was four years old, we came to this area around Gilroy—*la costa,* we called it—and worked in the fields here. We all worked in the fields as soon as we were able to walk and carry a bucket. I was picking prunes by the time I was five years old. We picked everything—garlic, onions, string beans, peaches, apricots, tomatoes, lettuce, sugar beets. We lived in camps and garages; when we lived in garages we also lived with rats. We were only free of rats when we camped out.

And always we lived with pesticides. Those toxins were poured on us. I can remember as a child working in the fields and watching the cute little planes come and fly over us. They flew so low that we could see the pilots in the little windows above the dust which came from the planes. We used to wave to the pilots, and we were delighted when they waved back to us.

We often had skin rashes as kids. My mother thought the rashes were from the sulphur which covered the tomato plants. Maybe they were. Maybe not. I also remember the yellow powder which covered the plants and was supposed to make them grow. We would get covered with it during the days we spent on our knees thinning out the young plants, and when the fields were watered, the water running from the rows of plants was yellow.

It was a typical farmworker's life. When I was thirteen years old we moved to the San Joaquin Valley, California's main agricultural region, where we picked grapes and cotton. I tell people that I have traveled from here to Madera and back either on my knees or on my butt.

I was still working in the fields when I got married. After we were married, my husband and I went to Delano to pick grapes. I got pregnant, had my first child, and then we moved back into this area. I started working in the cannery, where I stayed for twelve years. I wasn't being sprayed with pesticides within the walls of the cannery, but the tons of fruits and vegetables pouring into those canneries are covered with poison. When I had my last child I stopped working in the cannery, and then I worked as a housecleaner for pay.

In the late 1960s I began looking at my life and the lives of those around me with a more questioning eye. I enrolled in adult education classes for a year, and then I went to the community college. Those experiences opened up my world, and I began to understand more of who I am and what my role in this life is to be. That's when I first became involved in the community.

I was working with the Watsonville cannery workers strike* when I got sick. I was completely involved in that struggle, day and night. The strikers were 90 percent women, and they kept that strike going; whenever I went to the picket lines, there were the women, holding the fort. That strike was a national and international concern; even Jesse Jackson came to speak to the strikers. The strike also became a central issue for the whole Chicano community, and working with the strikers was a way for us to heighten public awareness of working conditions for Chicano women. Through that struggle we were able to bring to light many injustices, like the fact that there were no Chicanos on the school board or the city council, even though 80 percent of the population was Latino. We knew that if the Watsonville workers could win their fight, then we could address other problems like the terrible imbalance on the school board and the city council. So we supported the strike with everything we had.

While I was working with the strikers, I began to notice that I wasn't feeling very well. My life had been very hectic, but I did notice that I was losing weight. At first I thought the weight loss was just because I was running around so much and not paying attention to what I was eating. But I was also feeling a lot of discomfort in my stomach and then pain in my chest. I found I was walking around with my fist pressed against my breastbone because the pressure of my fist seemed to ease the pain a bit.

But I was so involved in the work of the strike that there was no room in my life for anything else. I felt I was fighting for our very survival, and I didn't have time to think about myself. Sometimes other people would tell me that I should slow down a bit

* On September 9, 1985, 1,100 workers, who were members of the International Brotherhood of Teamsters Local 912, began an eighteen-month strike against the Watsonville Canning Company over the issues of wages and benefits. The company wanted to lower their hourly wage of $6.66 to $4.25, take away many of their benefits (like medical insurance), and discontinue recognition of their union. The strike was finally settled on March 11, 1987. The workers won a three-year contract, maintenance of all their benefits and recognition of their union, even though Watsonville Canning Co. had been bought out by another company during the strike. The strikers suffered a 17 percent loss in wages, though this loss was much less than the company had wanted.

and take care of myself, but there was so much to do. There were many other people working with the strikers, of course, but I felt that I absolutely had to continue working because this struggle of the Watsonville strikers was so much a part of me. I had been a cannery worker; I knew exactly what these women were going through.

By the end of the strike, however, I finally had to admit that I was really sick. I was one of the principal organizers of the victory celebration in the San Jose union hall. My memory of the whole celebration is like that of a dream. I know that people talked to me and that I answered, but the only thing I remember saying was that any money we earned was to go to the committee of strikers. I was the last one there that night, cleaning up and packing my car. Then I went home and slept for the better part of two days.

Still, I felt exhausted. Now that my work with the strikers was completed, I had time to really acknowledge what I was feeling. I was in pain and my clothes hung on me. When I finally weighed myself, I discovered that I had lost nearly forty pounds. I decided that I had better see a doctor.

I went to my general practitioner, a doctor I trusted mostly because she was a woman. I described my symptoms to her and she decided on the basis of what I told her that I had arthritis in my breastbone. I was a little surprised, because there had been no history of arthritis in my family, but I agreed to take the medication she gave me.

The pain didn't go away, and I kept on losing weight. I went back to the doctor and this time she came up with a different diagnosis; this time, I think, she told me that she thought I had gas and she directed me to take antacids. I did as she said, but I was still vomiting whenever I ate. Then she took stool cultures, and when those proved to be clear of any infection, she told me that I should keep on taking the antacids. Over the next eight months, I went back seven times to see this physician. Each time, she gave me a different diagnosis and a different medication. One medication she prescribed gave me such a severe rash that she sent me to see a dermatologist who acted as though I were some sort of vermin; when I walked in the door of his office, he backed away and refused to touch me. Still I kept on believing in my physician. And I kept on losing weight.

Finally, one of my daughters told me that I had to demand an

X-ray of my stomach. I just was not getting better. I was getting sicker and sicker, my daughter said, and it was time for me to take charge.

My daughter was right. A barium X-ray of my stomach showed that there was something there, and I was immediately scheduled for a biopsy.

My whole family went with me—my children, their spouses and their children. That's a lot of people. The biopsy was a terrible experience. Some sort of tube was shoved down my throat into my stomach—an awful, awful sensation. After the biopsy, the doctor told me that I would need surgery right away, and then he went to talk to my family while I got dressed.

I was relieved; if the cancer could be taken care of by surgery, then I could get well. But my family seemed terribly depressed. We had a huge spaghetti dinner that night, and the house was full to overflowing with people. Everybody seemed determined to have a good time; still, I couldn't help but feel that all the gaiety was a bit forced. I couldn't eat, of course, and then I noticed that now and then someone would disappear outside. When they came back they looked as though they had been crying.

Something was wrong. I left the party early with the excuse that I was tired. The next morning I called one of my daughters and a granddaughter into my kitchen, sat them at the table, and told them I had something to say to them. "This is my body," I said, "and there is something going on here that I don't know about. I know you know what that is, and now you have to tell me—I want to understand my own body."

They told me. The doctor who had taken the biopsies had informed my family that I might not survive this cancer. He said that the surgeon might well open me up and then just close me up again. I was very upset that my family had been told something which had been kept hidden from me.

The next day I had an appointment with the surgeon. Again, my whole family went with me. The poor doctor was intimidated by the presence of so many people, and asked if I would choose only a few family members to include in the consultation. I answered that it shouldn't matter to him that there were so many people there. "You are not going to be talking to them," I said. "You are going to be talking to *me*. If any of my family have questions, then you can answer them. But you are talking to me, and at every point in my relationship with you, I am going to be the one making the decisions. I am a woman, and I know that it is my right to control my body."

The doctor's response was wonderful. He did talk to me. This time nothing was said behind my back. He also told me that he didn't think the cancer was as advanced as the doctor who had taken the biopsies had insinuated to my family.

Three days later I was in surgery. I was in the hospital for eleven days. People were with me constantly. The nurses complained that I wasn't getting enough rest. I did, of course. I slept while I had visitors, but there was hardly a minute when people weren't with me.

That was nearly two years ago. I'm not sick any longer, but I am not over that experience. I still suffer, though I no longer have pain in my stomach. I went through hell when I thought I was going to die, and the doubt is still there. Every time I return to the doctor for follow-up tests, I am afraid that he will find the cancer has returned. Sometimes I start crying and feeling sorry for myself, and I hate self-pity. But I never know when the cancer might come back. I am always preparing to die, always checking to be sure all my affairs are in order, and always trying to think of ways to pass on what I know to my children. I'm terrified still of other people's death, and I can't go to funerals. Sometimes when I am quiet, even sometimes when I am watching television, I will suddenly feel myself tighten up and find I am clenching my fists. The fear has never left me. My God, I say to myself, I have had cancer. Doesn't anyone understand that I had cancer? Cancer changes you.

Though I am afraid, I am also angry. I am always thinking about where this cancer might have come from. A few years back there was a lot of malathion sprayed to kill a fruit fly invasion in this area. Who knows what that might do to us? We are living in a society which is full of filth, filth that is making us sick, filth that made me sick, filth that made my family and my community sick. And they try to tell us it's our fault. We are not the ones making money out of the toxic materials being dumped on us or put in our food and our meat. If we are not the ones making the money, why should we accept the blame for our illnesses? Who is it that makes the money? They are the ones to blame—the rich, the corporations, and the government which helps the corporations make that money.

Many of us who must sell our physical labor in order to sur-

vive—especially we who are minorities—are still living and working in hazardous, unhealthy conditions. We will continue to get
cancer and other terrible diseases in a greater proportion than
those in the white society who are able to escape unsafe and
injurious environments. Farmworkers continue to work amid
poisons, and the fields of California have developed towns which
are "cancer clusters" where most of the cancers are leukemias
taking the lives of farmworker children.

The surgeon who removed my stomach told me once that in
this country Latinos and Japanese people have a greater proportion
of stomach cancer than other ethnic groups. When I think about
it, that's not so surprising. The Japanese, of course, are also
immigrants who have traditionally worked in the fields of California.

Before the United Farmworkers began organizing in the agricultural fields, poor, rural, and largely itinerant farmworkers didn't
have medical care. We didn't see doctors. If many of the farmworkers had died of cancer, no one would know because those deaths
would never have been documented and would never have been
factored into any statistical study. My maternal grandmother, for
instance, who worked in the fields all her life, died from what
we called a "dropped womb." She died at home under the care
of a *curandera*, who treated her with herbs and things like that.
All we knew was that her insides were diseased.

My great aunt lost five young daughters in two and a half
years—they had all been working in the fields. No autopsy was
ever performed, and we do not know what killed them. Other
members of my family, under the care of only a *curandera*, have
died at home from undiagnosed illnesses. What caused their deaths
will never be known. Likewise, we have no way of knowing how
many undocumented farmworkers who have come to the fields
from Mexico were harmed by the pesticides. Before the amnesty
program, thousands of those workers who lived and worked in
the fields—some of them for years—were deported every day.
We know nothing about what happened to them.

In more recent years there have been numerous studies about
the relationship of pesticide use to the high incidence of cancer
in farmworker communities. To date, the medical authorities and
government agencies say they cannot conclusively establish a
causal relationship. We who have lived our lives in the fields and
have suffered those illnesses need no further proof. And as the

poisonous pesticides continue accumulating in the bodies not just of the farmworkers, but also of the consumers who never even see the fields, perhaps there will finally be a movement of people large enough to force the big growers and their government protectors to grow healthy food, not just profitable food.

I am not religious, but I have some good friends who are priests. When I was sick they were with me all the way. I have a button that reads, "The more you complain, the more God lets you live." Before I had the surgery, I showed that button to one of my priest friends, and I told him that I thought it was very true. "And I am going to tell you right now, Father," I said, "that if there is a God and a Heaven, and if I go there and see Peter or Paul or whoever it is that stands at the gates, and if I see people still waiting to get in, I am going to demand that those doors be opened! If those doors aren't opened immediately, I am going to bring up banners and begin to organize, especially if those people are minorities!" The priest laughed. "I don't doubt it," he said. "I don't doubt that you will do just that."

Mother's Milk— as Safe as Apple Pie?

LISA GAYLE

When the telephone rang that early spring morning, I was not prepared for my friend's question. "Did you see the paper? That incinerator is going to be built practically in your back yard." I unfolded the *Detroit Free Press*; across the front page the headline proclaimed, "Trash plant raises cancer risk."[1]

It was almost three years since my cancer had been diagnosed and excised. At thirty-three I had been an invincible youth; overnight I became middle-aged. I was wary. My doctor told me that my chances of developing another cancer were six times higher than the chances of those who never had the disease. I made the changes that shaken survivors make to increase our odds for health: I changed my diet and I became serious about meditation and psychotherapy.

But the front page of the newspaper made it clear to me that my chances of forestalling another tumor did not depend solely on lifestyle.

The city of Detroit doesn't think of itself as being in the business of causing cancer, but like most cities, Detroit disposes of its garbage in huge pits called landfills. Landfill space is running out. As an alternative, the proposed incinerator plant would burn the city's garbage and use a portion of that energy for heat. In the process, however, it would violate Federal Clean Air regulations and add to the greenhouse effect by spewing lead, mercury, and thousands of tons of acid rain-causing gases into the air. As a survivor of cancer, I was most shaken by the knowledge that this plant would produce dioxin.

Dioxin appears to be one of the most toxic of manmade chemical compounds. The culprit in Agent Orange, dioxin can damage the liver and kidneys, interfere with the body's ability to fight infection, depress the immune system, and cause cancer. It does this destruction with amounts so tiny that the chemical is measured in parts per trillion.

It was no accident that the poisonous dioxin-producing trash plant was to be built in my back yard. My neighborhood on the east side of Detroit had been battered for years. In the fifties it was divided in half to make room for an interstate highway. In 1980 Chrysler shut down its oldest assembly plant, and a major source of employment left the area. Shortly after, 1,400 homes were razed by the city, and the land was practically given to General Motors for the building of an assembly plant which has provided no new employment. By 1986, a once stable, integrated, working-class neighborhood had become dotted with burnt houses, empty lots and stripped cars. Crack roamed the alleys and school yards. The infant mortality rate was the same as in Honduras.[2] And now we were to have a dose of dioxin.

I've had cancer once. I don't want it again. I joined the fight to stop the incinerator.

Three months after the announcement about the plans to build the incinerator, we read the startling results of a recent study. Dr. Arnold Schecter, Professor of Preventive Medicine at the State University of New York at Binghamton, conducted the study, which revealed that "An infant who is breast-fed for one year receives more dioxin than the dose many government agencies permit in a lifetime."[3]

Dioxin. A known cancer-causing agent. In mother's milk.

Great concern spread among my women friends. Thinking they were doing the best they could for their children, some of my friends were breast-feeding. Now these women began to doubt the wisdom of that decision. We eagerly awaited more information. La Leche League and the EPA reassured mothers, but no further articles followed the Schecter announcement. News which should have provoked a full-scale discussion was effectively diffused by a blackout of information.

I felt much like I had when my chondrosarcoma was taken out and my hip replaced. No one told me then that I would spend the next three months in a wheelchair, that my foot would be paralyzed, that the operation would affect my ability to walk and stand. I did not have the chance to make an informed decision about my surgery, yet I must live with the disability.

I have learned from having cancer. I am more skeptical of doctors; neither an "expert" nor the government has the right to decide what happens to my life. I know that we live with risk every day and that not all choices are easy ones. But whether we are making decisions about a cancer treatment, breast-feeding our children, or taking a plane ride, we are entitled to the information available. It is both our right and our responsibility to be educated and to make informed decisions.

No one set out to make dioxin. It is produced as a result of burning substances (like plastic) which contain chlorine. It is found in auto exhaust, used auto oil, some herbicides (like Agent Orange), wood preservatives, and more recently in bleached paper products. It has found its way into our food, water, and air.

It has not always been there. Dioxin comes from fairly recent industrial processes. On Isle Royale, a wilderness island in Lake Superior, dioxins were absent from sediments until about 1940. Their presence increases over the years.[4] Except for South Vietnam, which was covered with Agent Orange, in non-industrial countries the levels of dioxin are very low. In industrial countries, the levels are much higher.

Dioxin has been found in more than 400 consumer products, including 2-, 4-, 5-T, Silvex, Kuron, Weed-be-gone, and similar weed killers.[5] Some of these products are being withdrawn from the market. Due to the protests led by women whose children had been born with birth defects in Humboldt County, California in 1979, the EPA gained a suspension of spraying with these products around highway right-of-ways and forests.[6]

The largest source of dioxin now appears to be incineration. Because incineration plants burn waste, including paper and plastic, incineration creates dioxin. In the new generation of incinerators, which burn at very high temperatures in an attempt to destroy toxic chemicals, dioxin is still created as the ash cools off.[7]

We don't know how much exposure to dioxin is too much, nor do we know the effect of dioxin in combination with other toxic chemicals. According to Barry Commoner, there is considerable evidence that dioxins act as cancer promoters.[8] They don't change the genetic structure in the cells, but once these changes are caused by other chemicals, cancer promoters encourage the formation of tumors.

Dioxin is stored primarily in the fatty tissues of the body, containing the chemical and keeping it away from the blood, liver, or kidneys where it could do much more harm. A nursing mother, however, mobilizes her stores of fat to create milk. With that milk comes dioxin.

With the participation of twelve European countries and research groups in the United States and Canada, the World Health Organization (WHO) Regional Office for Europe has been coordinating studies on dioxins in human milk. They have reached an interim assessment of the risk to the health of infants.

A child's exposure starts in the uterus. The exposure increases during breast-feeding and then through eating food. The amount of exposure during a nursing period of six months is less than 5 percent of the amount a person might receive during her lifetime.[9] Yet during these six months the amount of exposure received by an infant is a concentrated one.

Like an adult, an infant accumulates dioxin in fatty tissue. But unlike an adult, during those first six months the infant puts on a lot of fat. Dr. Renatta Kimbrough of the Environmental Protection Agency (EPA), and a former participant in the WHO project, says that the gain in fat dilutes the toxin so that the concentration isn't greater than when the child was born. But after six months an infant puts on less fat, and this change in growth would increase the concentration of dioxin in the infant's tissues.[10] However, during these first six months of breast-feeding, the amount of dioxins in the mother decreases, though what this change indicates about the concentration of dioxin in her child's tissues if she continues to breast-feed is unclear.

The WHO and Dr. Kimbrough recommend that despite the presence of chemicals in human milk, breast-feeding should be encouraged and promoted on the basis of convincing evidence that the benefits of human milk to the overall health and development of an infant outweigh the risks. They estimate that a baby nursing for six months receives one-tenth to one-thousandth the amount of toxins necessary to cause adverse effects.[11]

Dr. Schecter disagrees. While not willing to tell all women not to breast-feed, he leans toward high quality formulas. "I don't know if mothers should breast-feed. There won't be an answer for a few years, and that will be different depending on the alternatives. For the middle class with access to sterile, high quality formulas, that might be the way to go. For poorer mothers, it's a real problem. They don't have that option."[12]

I have spent a long time trying to decide whether or not I should breast-feed. There is no good answer. What is clear is that one of the primary acts of human bonding, providing nurturance and sustenance, carries with it toxic chemicals. Why aren't there better answers?

Although dioxin causes liver cancer in rats, some scientists are hesitant to link dioxin with cancer in people because they say we may be less sensitive than rats. Decreased human sensitivity to some chemicals has been demonstrated, but also great errors have been made in underestimating a risk. Thalidomide was safe when tested on hamsters; humans are seven hundred times more sensitive to that particular drug.

Compounding the difficulties in establishing risk from exposures to toxic agents is the fact that cancers can take forty years to develop. In 1971, in Times Beach, Missouri, for example, the roads were oiled with a mixture that contained dioxin. People began to sicken. In 1983, the town was evacuated and the residents relocated. Times Beach is now closed down; even its exit sign was removed from the interstate highway. It's too early to tell if people from Times Beach will develop more cancers, but they are being watched. Doctors have already found a decrease in their immune systems' ability to function.[13] We are learning from AIDS patients that problems with the immune system can lead to cancer as well as other illnesses, but we may not see the full effect on the people from Times Beach for many years.

Not only does the length of time between exposure to carcinogenic chemicals and the development of cancers make proving the connection difficult, but the demands of the "scientific method" make unequivocal proof nearly impossible. If we want to demonstate the effect of small amounts of dioxin on people, it is important that studies contrast a group affected by small amounts with a group not exposed at all. But, as the entire population of the United States is contaminated, how can we distinguish between dioxin-related and other illnesses?

The chemicals have powerful defenders. Dow Chemical, the manufacturer of Agent Orange, conducted a study which showed no increase in disease among workers exposed to dioxin. Dow Chemical's researchers used a routine series of tests not designed for measuring the types of defects that indicate a developing cancer. The study lasted for only two years, and it did not include workers who might have become ill and left the company or workers who might have developed illnesses after retiring. Further, the control group was composed of men at Dow who had been exposed to many other chemicals.[14] Dow violated basic rules for scientific studies. Such sloppy research interferes with obtaining a realistic assessment of the effects of dioxin.

Our ability to identify carcinogens is far behind our ability to proliferate them; it is not surprising that more is not known about the risks of breast-feeding. Dioxin is not the only toxic chemical stored in the fat and mobilized during nursing. Aldrin, a pesticide once used for protecting corn crops, still persists in the soil. Chlordane, also used for corn, termites, and in the home, was banned after the EPA re-examined laboratory slides from studies which first reported the chemical to be non-carcinogenic. Lidane is used in flea bombs and Kwell shampoo, and as a fumigant for protecting seeds. PCBs and DDT, now banned, still accumulate in fat.

Whether they come through mothers' milk, infected food, contaminated water or polluted air, toxic chemicals pass into our children even before they are born. Cancer rates—particularly among children—are increasing. The scientists cannot give us satisfactory answers. What will we do about toxic, synthetic chemicals in the environment? Dr. Irving Selikoff comments, "These are no longer scientific problems. They are social problems, they are political problems, and they are problems in which the scientist can only make a contribution, which, however necessary, is not sufficient."[15]

Prevention is our key. Reducing the input of these chemicals into the environment is the most effective way of limiting exposure to them. On this point the WHO and Drs. Commons, Kimbrough and Schecter all agree.

There are saner ways to deal with garbage. We can reduce the amount we make by not selling items by their packaging. We in the United States produce twice as much garbage per person as do the Europeans. Making plastics creates toxic waste. We can substitute other products for much of the plastic we use; the widespread use of plastics is only forty years old. We can reuse what we have; garbage does not cease to exist when we throw it away. As a last resort, we can recycle. Recycling is much more effective if it is done by an entire community. We need to separate our recylables in our homes and have them collected at the curbside with what is left of our garbage. Yet this simple and effective effort to reduce our enormous amounts of waste has been organized in very few communities in the United States.

The current trend in handling waste is not toward prevention; rather, we appear to be increasing pollution. A study reported in a Long Island newspaper disclosed that while state governments have spent $300 million promoting incineration, only $8 million was spent on promoting recycling.[16] Many communities are facing the exhaustion of landfill space. Over two hundred incineration plants are slated to be constructed in the United States,[17] and almost half of all solid waste may be incinerated by the middle of the 1990s. The ash produced by incineration is toxic. Dioxin, created in the stacks, will escape into the air or be buried in landfills that eventually leak into our water supply.

The government cooperates with the trend toward pollution. EPA studies of the health threat from dioxins produced by incineration only take into account what is inhaled; they ignore other ways in which dioxin enters the human body. The 1988 EPA budget for garbage and other "non-hazardous" waste programs is 2 percent of what it was in 1980. Although mandated by Congress to find solutions, the EPA has not formulated guidelines to regulate incinerator ash.

The handling of waste is big business these days. The company which is the builder of Detroit's incinerator, along with many other companies, has little or no experience in building or operating a new generation of incinerators; the technology is untested. That Detroit company used to build nuclear power plants. Their background does not inspire confidence.

In the winter of 1989 workers in the Detroit incinerator became ill when exposed to the ash. They walked off the job twice. A sample of ash was tested by Greenpeace and found to have 800 times enough lead and 200 times enough cadmium to classify it as a hazardous substance.[18] The ash was not tested for dioxin. This ash is now dumped in a non-hazardous waste landfill in a rural community near Detroit.

Residents in that community are angry; they have joined thousands in Detroit who are opposed to the incinerator. Dozens have been arrested during protests, and Detroit juries have not convicted any of them. In Windsor, the Canadian city across the Detroit River, the City Council collected 39,000 signatures—one-quarter of the population—in a petition drive to oppose the incinerator. Native Americans from Walpole Island, located in the Detroit River between the United States and Canada, see the incinerator as another encroachment on their lives, and they, too, have joined the fight.

Detroit residents are not alone. Washington, D.C.'s incinerator ash lies next to a basketball court owned by St. Elizabeth's psychiatric hospital. In Minneapolis, Minnesota, and Austin, Texas, residents are fighting to stop incinerators. In Brooklyn, New York, they have succeeded. Other governments are facing problems in getting rid of the ash. In 1988 a shipload of toxic waste from Philadelphia toured the Third World with not a single country willing to accept the waste. The ship was filled with incinerator ash.

There is no way to escape the poison. Nevertheless, there are some precautions which new mothers can take against passing to their babies the dioxin accumulated in their bodies. Reducing intake of food from high on the food chain, in which the levels of contamination are more concentrated, can help. Avoiding freshwater fish and emphasizing high fiber foods like grains, fresh fruits and vegetables (well washed) can help. Nursing women should not try to lose weight while they are breast-feeding, as excessive weight reduction might mobilize more toxins from the fat stores. In addition, there appears to be less dioxin passed to a second child if the first child has been breast-fed.

The half life of dioxin in the body is about five years. That is, in five years half of the dioxin that is consumed or breathed in today will be gone from the body. It is eliminated in the feces. There is currently no generally accepted method for hastening this elimination process, though the Japanese are conducting experiments to determine if charcoal or other substances can increase the body's elimination of dioxin.

Of all the effects on the human body from the barrage of toxic elements which we cannot escape, cancer is the most insidious. No matter how close any of us is to another person, no matter how warmly we are held or how many shoulders we have to cry on, the fight with cancer goes on in our bodies, and it makes each of us feel very much alone. Still, many of us respond to having cancer with tremendous strength and courage. We fight for our lives, surprising ourselves at our own capabilities. We get angry at God, or the doctor, or both. We accept living with illness, disability, death.

But cancer is a social disease. Society has made a decision: we tolerate an increasing number of early, painful and expensive deaths because we choose to stick our heads in the sand each time the connection between synthetic chemicals and the increasing rates of cancer is made.

We must look. If we are even considering that mother's milk is now carcinogenic, the stakes are too high. I wonder when we will face how overwhelming the reality is, how big a fight we have ahead of us, and how desperately we need to band together. If the WHO is right—that is, if the amount of dioxin a nursing infant now receives is one-tenth to one-thousandth of the amount that will cause ill effects—it is not too late to act.

NOTES

1. *Detroit Free Press*, April 4, 1986.
2. Dzwonkowski, Ron, "State to Fight Infant Deaths," *Detroit Free Press*, January 30, 1984, Section A, p. 3.
3. Telephone interview with Dr. Arnold Schecter, Department of Preventive Medicine, State University of New York, Clinical Campus at Binghamton, August 14, 1987.
4. Czaczwa, Jean, Bruce McVeety, Ronald Hites, "Polychlorinated Dibenzo-p-dioxins and Dibensofurans in Sediments from Siskiwit Lake, Isle Royale," *Science*, November 2, 1984, p. 568.
5. Samuels, Mike, M.D. and Hal Zina Bennett, *Well Body, Well Earth: Health Source Book*, Sierra Club Books, 1983, p. 153.
6. Samuels, p. 153.
7. Commoner, Barry, "Incinerators: The City's Half-Baked and Hazardous Solution to the Solid-Waste Problem," *New York Affairs*, Vol. 9, No. 2, 1985, p. 29.
8. Commoner, p. 22.
9. Results of Analytical Field Studies on Levels of PCBs, PCDDs, and PCDFs in Human Milk, Report on a WHO Consultation, Copenhagen, Feb. 24-25, 1988, p. 4.
10. A telephone interview with Renatta Kimbrough on August 12, 1987.
11. Results of Analytical Field Studies on Levels of PCBs, PCDDs, and PDDFs in Human Milk, Report on a WHO Consultation, Copenhagen, February 24-25, 1988, p. 5.
12. Telephone interview with Dr. Arnold Schecter, August 14, 1987.
13. Hoffman, Richard E., P.A. Stehr-Green, K.B. Webb, et. al., "Health Effects of Long Term Exposure to 2, 3, 7, 8-tetrachlorodibenzo-p-dioxin," *Journal of the American Medical Association*, April 18, 1986, p. 2013.
14. Selikoff, Irving J., "Lessons for Living in a Chemical World," *Bulletin of Environmental Contamination Toxicology*, 1984, p. 694.
15. Selikoff, p. 695.
16. Murtagh, Connie, "Recycling: Waste as Resource," *Greenpeace*, Vol. 13, No. 13, p. 10.
17. Christrup, Judy, "Rising From the Ashes: Our Trash Shouldn't Burn," *Greenpeace*, Vol. 13, No. 3, p. 8.
18. *Evergreen Alliance Newletter*, February, 1989, p. 5. This was a sample of ash smuggled out of the incinerator by concerned workers and handed to Greenpeace activists who performed the test.

Exposure

SUSAN EISENBERG

When that same question lunged at her
again, a second doctor asking: have you
ever been exposed to
radiation? a whirl of random images began
flashing in steady rotation—

    milk with strontium 90

    X-rays for bronchitis

    working at MIT: yellow barrels
    marked with nuclear symbols/
    rooftop vents she was warned to
    stay clear of

Was she among those who breathed
Chernobyl/Three Mile Island/or
other accidents, unreported? was the
playground where she skipped rope
a waste dump, disguised?

    plates of fish she has eaten

    walks along abandoned railroad tracks

    every inhale/every taste/every
    open skin pore now suspect

Who on this planet could
answer such a question
asked, so nonchalantly, with anything but
Yes or
Not that I know of.

There is so much we are not told.

The Story of a Downwinder

ZINNA EPPERSON

In April of 1986, the Chernobyl accident shocked the whole world. That same year in the United States, the Department of Energy was forced under the Freedom of Information Act to release documents which revealed that the Hanford nuclear complex in the state of Washington had pumped over a million curies of radioactive iodine into the air and tens of billions of gallons of radioactive waste into the ground, much of which seeped into the beautiful Columbia River. The largest single emission from Hanford was a secret and deliberate one on December 2, 1949, when 7,780 curies of radioactive iodine-131 and 20,000 curies of zenon-133 were released,[1] a discharge many hundreds of times larger than the Three Mile Island nuclear accident in 1979 which resulted in a seven-fold increase in infant mortality in that area.[2] My life and the lives of thousands of other people who lived near the Hanford plants have been seriously affected. "Those dangers to health and life are still occurring today . . . and their effects will become manifest over many years to come. The map of the United States is, in effect, studded with radioactive and toxic Department of Energy footprints on the future."[3]

Two decades before the truth about Hanford was to surface, I moved to Kennewick, Washington, downwind from Hanford, with my husband and my six-month-old daughter. I was twenty that hot summer day in 1966, and it was an exciting time for me. My husband of one year was taking us to his childhood home. I would meet his family for the first time. I had no idea what to expect, and my heart sank when I first viewed the Horse Heaven Hills. So this is what he meant by "dry land farming." The whole place looked like a desert with its dry, dusty browns and golds. I thought hills should have trees and streams and wildlife, so I was very relieved to discover that his family home was by the Columbia River.

My sister-in-law, Joyce, who had the first goiter I'd ever seen, filled me in on the family history. Among her stories there was her own history of strange illnesses and miscarriages. And there was a story about Willy who died at age four with stomach cancer. There were stories about Linda, an eight-year-old child of a nearby family friend, who lost her hair and eyelashes. Her hair grew back, but not her eyelashes. The doctor said she was "emotional." But I was strong and healthy and eager to get on with life. I intended to add my share to this already large clan. I've always loved challenges, and I quickly adjusted to the fantastic wind storms that could turn a loaded semi completely around. It was a challenge to grow food with little water, to can food and grow grains for cereals and bread. l loved it, and best of all was the refreshing swim in a lagoon which was a quarry pit now filled with cool Columbia River waters, a popular swimming and fishing spot.

But after that first year the dream began to twist out of shape. My hair would suddenly fall out in chunks and then grow back. "Probably nerves," the doctors told my husband. I became pregnant easily and often, only to miscarry at three months or give birth at six or seven months. "You are too high strung," I was told, and my violent attacks of nausea were cited as proof. When I experienced unexplained exhaustion or illness, the doctors told my husband I was looking for attention. Over the next few years my marriage slowly became a nightmare in a world made up of a resentful husband, piling medical bills, and premature babies born dead or dying of cranial hemorrhaging.

Four years after I had married, I was a divorced mother of two. My second living child was a boy who had extreme allergies the first two years of his life. As he grew older his allergies improved, but he was almost totally deaf due to thick scar tissue covering both eardrums. He also became increasingly crippled as he grew because his leg tendons were not growing with him. In the first of sixteen moves over the next thirteen years—constant attempts to find better medical care, better income, and more tolerance for my Native American heritage—I moved to Oregon in 1970. Our health did seem to improve in Oregon, but I could not make ends meet on welfare there. We needed the support of a family. Since I was an orphan, the only family available to us were my ex-in-laws, and so I returned to Kennewick.

For a while all seemed well, and I was able to move into low income housing. The family of my ex-husband was as supportive as I had hoped, and I became active in politics, pushing for equal treatment for fixed-income people. Subsequently, I remarried and moved to California.

The birth of my ninth child, a daughter conceived in California, was full-term and uneventful, and while our family was very poor, we were very happy. Then on Christmas Eve, my second husband had a car accident. He suffered a minor head injury, but no matter what we tried, we were unable to completely stop the wound from bleeding. Finally, we sold everything and returned to Oregon with the hopes that we could find medical care for him there.

During the move back to Oregon I also learned I was expecting again. I blamed stress for the return of thinning hair, extreme nausea and exhaustion. It was on the day of our first anniversary that my husband was taken home by his family to be cared for until he died. I suffered an agony of guilt and exhaustion, and that summer of 1972 remains a haze in my memory. My son was born prematurely with his lungs and liver not functioning properly, and he had cranial hemorrhaging. Like the others, this baby started having convulsions. But he was luckier than the others, all of whom had died. The doctors were able to save this one.

Against my will, my first husband had taken our children away from me and had moved with them to California. I lost custody of my children because I was poor and in ill health, and also because I was an Indian who insisted on following the Native American religion. In Oregon during the 1970s I found attitudes towards Native Americans more tolerant, but California still disapproved of us and our customs and beliefs. I became involved for a short while with the American Indian Movement while I attended community college and became a peer counselor for Native Americans coming from Rosebud and other Dakota reservations. It was at this time that I began my fight with cancer, first of the cervix. My cervix was cauterized, and then I had to have a partial hysterectomy.

I was shocked and frightened when I first learned of my cervical cancer. My doctor comforted me by telling me that the cancer was not advanced and was most likely curable. With much relief I joked to the doctor that if his diagnosis were wrong and the cancer was more advanced that he had thought, he could go right ahead and remove my uterus. I would welcome protection from any more babies, I told him; too many of my babies had died already. My willingness, even apparent eagerness, to sacrifice future pregnancies shocked the doctor. Though he knew my history, he expressed holier-than-thou concern that any woman would be so willing to give up her uterus. Apparently contemplating the removal of a uterus is an acceptable notion only if it comes from the doctor.

As it turned out, I did have to have a partial hysterectomy. Shortly after the surgery I began experiencing symptoms of menopause, and when I complained about those symptoms, the doctor first tried to convince me that the symptoms were all in my imagination. Finally, however, I was given hormone therapy "to shut her up," as a nurse put it. The hormones did ease my symptoms, and though I felt angry and humiliated by my treatment, I also felt vindicated later when my own research confirmed that women who have partial hysterectomies do indeed experience a temporary reduction in hormonal activity.

Not long after the hysterectomy, I found a lump under my arm. The doctor reacted with considerable alarm and insisted that I have the lump removed immediately because, he said, I now had cancer in my lymph nodes. For the first time I became truly afraid for my life. No one could explain why I should suddenly be developing tumors, but I knew now that my battle for health and life was going to be a very serious one. I was terrified for my children from my second marriage, whom I still had with me, for who would raise them if cancer took my life? I had certainly had problems in the past with my health, but now I truly began to realize my own mortality. And I began to doubt my ability to care for myself and my children.

In my frantic search for a means of survival for myself and my children, I turned to various social agencies for help. I found neither help nor encouragement. Rather, I was confronted with condemnation for being both poor and ill; I was a double failure. I'll never forget waking up in the hospital after one cancer removal to find welfare people shoving papers under my nose, demanding that I "think of the children and sign these papers" releasing the children from my custody. I thank a friend who hid my children in her home until I was able to function again.

It was all too much and too overwhelming. Marriage seemed like the only way out. I got married for the third time, this time in an Indian ceremony, to a mixed-blood man who also had children. We moved to California, where my husband could continue his studies, and there we had to be married again by a justice of the peace; California did not recognize Indian religion, and I did not want to lose my children. Within four years I found myself divorced once again. My third husband had turned to drugs and alcohol to deal with our problems, and he beat me often. During those "battering years," as I think of them, I developed a tumor in one breast which had to be removed. There it was again—another tumor. In fear, I had kept the discovery of this tumor to myself, but the night before I was to be admitted to the hospital I finally told my husband, foolishly looking to him for comfort. He beat me so severely that the hospital had to delay the surgery until I had healed enough for the surgeon to clearly see the area of the tumor.

Many times I turned to the law for help, trying to seek protection from my battering husband. I would move away from him, only to come home from work and find him there. Because I could not save enough money for a divorce lawyer, and because there was no legal aid for the poor, and because the California laws did not protect abused wives, my husband apparently had every right to take my money and continue to move in on me whenever and wherever he found me. The state wanted to take my children away because they said I was too ill to properly care for them, and my son was becoming impossible to care for alone. In desperation I gave my last two children to my first husband to raise, signing adoption papers over to him. I was down to 102 pounds, had black bags under my eyes and a rash covering half my face. I could walk only with the greatest difficulty and extreme pain. Once again I took myself to Oregon and hid out with friends until my divorce was filed and finalized.

That same year, 1978, I had to contend with cancer again. This time I had thyroid surgery, and three "hot spots" were removed. I remember that I was in fine shape to answer the door that Halloween; the surgery scars were fresh and made a perfect addition to my scary costume.

I found that I could not live on my own with only the SSI payments, plus Medicaid and a few dollars in food stamps, so I moved to Redding, California, where SSI is double what I had received in Oregon. Still determined to work and receive an education, I helped start a battered women's shelter and worked the local crisis line. Through these two agencies I was able to receive college equivalency in psychology, specializing in suicide prevention, abuse and battering, and I worked as a welfare advocate. Then in 1980 the doctors discovered that I had systemic lupus, gave me six months to live, and put me on heavy doses of prednisone.

Since then, I have experienced a continuous decline in energy, strength, and ability. I have continued to get tumors, mostly benign, and I have developed chronic pancreatitis due to lupus attacks. I was forced to cut my beautiful long hair to minimize its thinness; I can no longer hold my arms up long enough to brush it, anyway. Because my body does not metabolize properly any more, I have chronic build-ups of calcium deposits in my knees and other joints. My spine continues to disintegrate, and I await neck surgery in hopes of recovering the use of my muscles, or at least slowing the progression of weakness and fatigue. These days it is very hard to walk any distance, type more than a few minutes at a time, exert the mild pressure it takes to use a pen or pencil, or drive very far. Doctors shake their heads over "strange" symptoms and multiple sclerosis-like reactions to radiation from the sun, electric heaters, light bulbs or temperatures over seventy-five degrees. I have difficulty performing tasks that were once easy, such as spelling or doing math, and I have memory lapses.

Of ten pregnancies (twelve babies), I have four surviving. All have degenerative spinal problems. My oldest daughter also has a huge optical pit, and, like me, has had cancer of the cervix. She has carried one child successfully, but she is experiencing some difficulty with her second pregnancy. My oldest son had surgery to correct his tendons, nicking them along their length to stretch them, and he has also had his ears repaired. My youngest daughter was diagnosed with cervical cancer at the age of eighteen; she continues to have spinal problems and may—again, like me— have a thyroid problem. My youngest son has short tendons, but he can keep them stretched with exercise. He also has continuing problems in other areas.

"Positive thinking" groups insisted that I really wanted to be ill when I failed to think myself well. Religious groups accused me of not trusting God when I failed to be miraculously cured. Mental health agencies told me that I harbored subconscious negative anger from my childhood because it was proven that negative emotions cause cancer. And welfare seemed more interested in taking my children away from me than in helping me raise them. With the "assistance" of those agencies, I felt useless and ashamed because I could no longer hold a paying job.

One evening a few years ago I turned on my television set, and suddenly the pieces of my life's puzzle—the patterns of illness and misery—fell into place. The show was "West 57th Street." I was tired that evening and not paying much attention to the television. Then I heard the names of Hanford and the Tri-Cities, and I began to listen. At first I sat there unbelieving as the story unfolded about the Hanford Nuclear Plant and how it has been contaminating the Tri-City area with iodine-131 and radiation. As I listened to descriptions of the health problems suffered by the Downwinder population, I flew back and forth between towering rage and soaring elation. Now I understood! Now there was finally a concrete reason for the cancers and other tumors, the lupus that didn't always fit the pattern, the many miscarriages, the infant deaths, and the health problems of my living children. Now maybe I could get some real help. Now that the truth was out, something would be done for people like me.

My exhilaration from this discovery was equalled only by my outrage. I listened first in paralyzed pain as I heard the show's host tick off a list of illnesses connected with radiation and iodine-133, and my mind jumped from one memory to another as I relived the cranial hemmorhaging, the seizures, the birth defects, the hormonal problems which had plagued me and my children. How often I had blamed myself! How often I had labeled myself as a "bad" mother, a "bad" wife. And all this time the real reasons for my troubles had been known by the plant and by our government. In fact, they had released the cloud of radiation on purpose, as an "experiment." The rage I felt was the dawn of my determination to learn more so that I could help to stop this cruel insanity.

Several doctors have expressed interest in the fact that I had been exposed to iodine-131 and radiation, and they tell me they suspect that the exposure might be the basic cause of my cancers and other myriad difficulties. I do have "blue-spotted DNA cells" which are consistent with radiation poisoning. But most doctors do not know anything about radiation poisoning, and I think they should be interested to learn at least some of what I have had to learn the hard way. The doctors, however, mostly appear disinterested and repeat to me that my case is too complicated. I am again resigned to being treated by physicians as a piecemeal object; the gynecologist treats the cystic ovaries, the spine surgeon looks at my spine, the eye doctor watches for cataracts. Until I was finally diagnosed as having a "legitimate" disease, one the doctors could put a name to, I felt that the doctors always dismissed me as a complainer. And since I am a woman it is easier for them to label me with that old designation of "nerves" or "female complaints." Some simply take the attitude that every problem is due to the lupus and so there is no use in doing anything, while others tell me I must "learn to live" with my difficulties, but they never say how.

I am still not able to get any medical insurance, and so I must remain on Medi-Cal, which makes it difficult for me to obtain adequate care. The doctors are not to blame for the fact that I must be on Medi-Cal, but I do blame our government. The government allows widespread pollution, covers up mistakes, pays off some radiation victims, and denies responsibility for others. Hanford, for instance, is protected from lawsuits; even though it has been disclosed that government technicians at Hanford secretly experimented on the surrounding population,[4] not many of that population are well enough to testify and hopefully be compensated for at least our medical expenses. I, for one, am no longer healthy enough to travel, nor do I have the means to go to meetings or court hearings, so I must rely on my typewriter and on other people to make my experience and what I feel about it known.

I think that our government needs to subsidize studies on iodine 131 and radiation poisoning effects. Doctors need to be taught how to recognize and treat such illnesses. We need doctors who specialize in radiation effects even to the fifth generation of those exposed. The nuclear plants like those at Hanford must be forced to accept responsibility and pay their victims, and they must pay to clean up their mess, the contamination of the surrounding lands and waters. Only in this way will they take active responsibility to *prevent* such wanton destruction of people, land, and resources.

NOTES

1. Steele, Karen Dorn, "1949 radiation release contaminated vast area," *The Spokesman-Review*, Spokane, Washington, May 4, 1989.
2. Wasserman, Harvey and Norman Solomon, et al., *Killing Our Own*, Dell Publishing Co., Inc., New York, 1982, pg. 251.
3. Statement by Physicians for Social Responsibility in an open letter sent to the White House in 1988.
4. Steele.

Numbers, Numbers, Numbers...

LOIS CAMP

I'm a third generation farm wife, and I've lived and worked in the country all my life. One morning in the fall of 1986, I found myself preparing to do something quite out of the ordinary for me. I was driving to Richland, Washington to testify before the Hanford Health Effects Panel, appointed by the Center for Disease Control (CDC) to hear public testimony and review 19,000 pages of recently released classified documents regarding the Hanford Nuclear site.

My mind bubbled over with questions. Would those experts listen to what I had to say? Would my testimony be effective? Would I present enough convincing information? Was I dressed appropriately? I reassured myself; I did not want to project an image which differed from who I really am—a rural woman who feels a deep obligation to defend her principles and who suspects that her people and her land had been grievously harmed. I never let my self-doubts stop me from relentlessly searching for the facts, and I would not let those doubts stop me now from telling the truth as I know it.

My story really begins many years ago when more than one million curies of radiation were released from the Hanford Nuclear Reservation between 1944 and 1956.[1] The truth about the radioactive emissions from Hanford did not surface until early in 1986, and, in fact, the whole truth is still seeping out piece by piece. Those of us living in the area knew that we were having more cancers—and other health problems—than other parts of the country. But we didn't know why.

I lived about fifty miles from the Hanford Reservation during my early childhood. In those early years I experienced health problems which I now believe can be attributed to my being dosed with radioactive emissions. My first hint of physical harm was a minor skin rash when I was eight or nine years old. But the rash didn't disappear as I had expected it to; it rapidly worsened, and within hours I became one mass of blisters which covered every inch of my body except for the soles of my feet. I ended up in the hospital, where for weeks I slid in and out of consciousness. My doctor was baffled.

I was given test after test, but all my doctor could say was that I had evidently come into contact with something so toxic that it had nearly killed me; he could not, however, determine what that toxic substance was. Ever since that time I have continued to have unusual skin disorders. I have a near-zero sun tolerance. My skin is easily irritated and infected, and it takes a very long time to heal.

The eruptions on my skin were only the beginning. I seem to have no resistance to infections, viruses, and fungi. At the age of forty-eight I have the energy level of an eighty-four-year-old; I've been recently diagnosed with cardiomyopathy (meaning that a major portion of my heart has been irreversibly damaged), and my doctor, one of the top cardiologists in the state, is stumped because he can't determine a cause for it. I had endometrial cancer in 1980 and then uterine cancer in 1983. Several members of my family have had cancer. Many of my friends have had (and died from) cancer. In fact, where we live cancer seems as prevalent as the common cold.

I first learned about the Hanford emissions from a newspaper article in the spring of 1986. Needless to say, I was stunned by the implications—for me and for my community—of this disclosure. I had a term paper due for a class I was taking, a perfect motive to find out more. I read articles and studies and statistics written by experts and specialists. But the more I read, the more muddled the "official" picture became.

The research I had done for my term paper provided me with enough information to seriously question many of the statistics I came across concerning numbers and percentages of cancer incidence and death, as well as the data on many other illnesses. Even at the very beginning of my study, I was amazed to learn that there were no actual 1986 population numbers available for local counties or school districts. The data from the 1980 census count was obtainable at the courthouse, but no one had any figures more current. I had hoped to find a baseline number of the actual population count so that the figures I had gathered about illnesses and deaths in those areas would yield fairly accurate percentage rates. It was curious, I thought, that so many other studies claimed to be accurate when the researchers couldn't have had recent population counts, either.

More reliable demographic data, however, doesn't insure officially sanctioned results. One example is the epidemiological study which was done in Garfield County (downwind of the Hanford plant). That county is largely agrarian with a relatively small population and low mobility, making its residents ideal for a study of long-term exposure to environmental hazards. Some health care providers in Pomeroy, the county seat, became concerned about the "very high"[2] cancer rate there, particularly the number of cases of pancreatic cancer in their area. In the early 1980s they had directed a study which verified causes of death, including examination of death certificates. In an effort to uncover what might lie behind the elevated cancer statistics for this community, Garfield County officials conducted a detailed analysis of numerous water sources in the county because water was the one element they could isolate as being common to all the people in the county. They found no significant levels of the pesticides or herbicides which had been the most widely suspected contaminants. This inconclusive investigation left the question of environmental factors in the pancreatic cancer rate unanswered. When the report about the Hanford emissions became public in 1986, it seemed evident that the area in which the cancers had occurred had undoubtedly received exposure to the radiation. The county had not had access to the equipment necessary to identify radioactive isotopes when the water analysis was done, and nobody was looking for radioactive isotopes, anyway. So the presence of this obvious carcinogenic agent remained unknown.

When legislators learned about the unresolved Garfield County study, they called a special public meeting. Officials from the Epidemiological Section of the Department of Social Health Services in Washington state, along with other high officials, were invited to attend. At the meeting, a Garfield County Health Department employee who had assisted in the earlier study of pancreatic cancer incidence was challenged by state health officials, as was the entire study.[3] The state officials insinuated the entire study lacked credibility. They implied that death certificates used may have been inaccurate as pancreatic cancer is difficult to diagnose, and the deceased may not have even had cancer!

The conjecture by health officials that death certificates might be imprecise intrigued me. What if they were right, and the death certificates really didn't accurately reflect the causes of death? If there was any doubt that death certificates were unimpeachable sources for information about causes of death, then certainly studies which depended upon them for any statistical analysis were seriously flawed. But what if the inaccuracy were the opposite of the accusation implied by the skeptics of the Garfield study? What if, in fact, some death certificates were inaccurately attributing causes of death to reasons other than cancer when cancer was the cause?

I began my own very unscientific and informal survey of illnesses and deaths in my rural school district area. One of my friends provided valuable information as she was a former city employee, and as part of her job had kept data on deaths for the last twenty-five years. In our school district alone, there had been an approximately 600 percent increase in stillbirths from 1961 to 1968. The actual numbers of total cases of stillbirths are considered "insignificant numbers" by the expert scientific researchers. I have often wondered if that's what they told the parents who are still suffering from their loss.

Another friend who was helping me compile a list of cancer deaths told me that she knew cancer was not listed on her father's death certificate, even though he had had cancer. He had died of organ failures which were listed on the death certificate form, but the cancer which had caused those organ failures was never mentioned. Time after time we encountered similar discrepancies between what people knew about a death and what appeared on the death certificate. But when I finally realized the full import of what we were accidentally discovering, I had no actual numbers to present to the panel. I had read numerous statistical studies about cancer and other disease incidence and deaths which were based on random selection of death certificates. If the death certificate omissions which my friend and I were uncovering represented even only a fraction of the death certificates used by other researchers, then their statistical conclusions would have to be skewed.

I recently spoke with a home health care nurse from our county who agrees with my rough estimate that cancer is evident in approximately 80 percent of the deaths in this area. In comparison, 22 percent of deaths nationally in 1987 were attributed to cancer. She is convinced that this area, at least, has a much higher number of cancer cases per capita than is statistically "normal." Not only are death certificates a questionable source on which to base a statistical study; another difficulty lies in the way in which data are gathered. Official statistics are "age-adjusted" so that, in essence, if a person is diagnosed with cancer after a certain age (such as seventy-five years), that cancer isn't included in the statistics. Presumably, the statisticians figure that the person would have died anyway from old age, and therefore the death is not statistically significant. So if eight out of ten of the cases which the nurse cared for were cancer, but three of those cancer cases were in older people, maybe only five of those would be credible statistical numbers. Many cancers take more than twenty years to develop after exposure to a carcinogenic substance. Discounting the cancer-related deaths of people over a certain age undermines the probability of statistics demonstrating that a particular area might suspect a specific contamination as being responsible for an abnormal increase in cancer cases. At best, these statistical maneuvers simply cloud the issue; at worst, they forestall people's efforts to understand and prevent the causes of a terrible disease.

Even with all the information I had at my command, I felt my knees quaking when my name was called to testify before the Hanford Health Effects Panel. After all, these people were the recognized experts in their fields; how could I expect them even to listen to an ordinary farm wife?

I had prepared my presentation much like I always did for a typical Sunday School or Bible School class. I had an enlarged map of eastern Washington on which I had highlighted all the areas I had lived in, and I had indicated the places where there were geographical clusters of illnesses. As I nervously moved into my testimony, I observed subtle changes in the panel members. Some sat up straight. Pencils stopped tapping. A few panel members began jotting notes. They were beginning to listen.

When I finished speaking, I turned to go back to my chair, still suspecting that there would be no response from the panel. To my surprise, one of the physicians began questioning me. First he requested that I provide him with more information about the study I had done. Then, almost defensively, he stated that he had never heard of a disease not being listed on a death certificate. I just shrugged my shoulders. I told him I didn't know about all death certificates, but I did know that the record of cancer as a primary cause for death had been left out of some death certificates here, and that if I could discover such omissions, there sure could be a chance that they happened elsewhere.

With a deep sigh of relief, I finally sat down. To my surprise, two newspaper reporters hurried to my side and began questioning me. At last it began to sink in; this farm gal just might have a story to share.

The slippery statistics, the cover-ups, and the deceptions which have historically provided a safety net for government agencies are sufficient reason to challenge the credibility of our official experts. A classic example of such bureaucratic duplicity appeared in an agricultural publication recently. The article hailed the studies done by a program of the United States Department of Agriculture (USDA) to measure erosion levels on the steep farm hills in our area. The USDA has given our local farmers an ultimatum to retard erosion unless they want to risk becoming ineligible for government programs like crop insurance, but many farmers have not been able to afford the expensive equipment and techniques required to prevent soil erosion. Now it appears that the USDA has a way of checking up on us. According to the article, they can measure the amount or depth of cesium-137 (Cs-137), which is a by-product of radioactive fission, in the soil at the top of a hill or from a flat area, and then measure the Cs-137 levels at the bottom of the hill. If there is more Cs-137 found in the soil samples from the bottom of the hill, they can conclude that there has been soil erosion. After nearly fifty years of being told that there was no "significant" contamination of radionuclides in our earth, that same authority (the U.S. government) can now announce that Cs-137 is not only present, but the presence is vast enough and consistent enough to be useful in a soil research program.[4]

The same article is careful not to implicate Hanford by maintaining that the Cs-137 in our area comes from the Nevada Test Site, despite the fact that we are behind the prevailing winds from the Test Site. But it doesn't really matter where the radioactive poison comes from. What's important is the fact that it's there at all. Cs-137 tends to travel to the bones when it enters a human body, and my first son has already had one bone tumor. Now I have learned that the soil on which he played as a child contains Cs-137, though all our questions about safety had only brought us emphatic reassurances that any contamination was so low that there could not be any ill effects on the population.

The personal and scientific data I have accumulated leads me to only one conclusion. I believe there has been a very real attempt, in the face of overwhelming evidence to the contrary, to discount environmental hazards as possible causes of cancer. The question we need to ask is: why? It is possible to expect the "experts" even to understand or care about our concerns? Can they imagine what it is like to learn that Cs-137 has been present in the dust that we have breathed all these years? Is this the price of progress? Is this what we are expected to pay for a strong defense?

I am no longer willing to let others answer these questions for me. My family has suffered from unusual cancers and other illnesses. I've had cancer twice myself. In frustration and desperation I pray that this insanity—the deceptions, contradictions, and denials—will stop. Since the 1986 acknowledgment of the Hanford releases, I have been on a merry-go-round; I always end up at the beginning instead of gaining any ground. No matter what information I present, there is always some "expert" with a briefcase full of numbers ready to contradict what I say. I have been reassured over and over again that our government will do everything they can and use every bit of information known in their assessment of health problems in our area, but nothing is ever specific. Generalizations and evasive double talk prevail.

I want to get off my merry-go-round. All of us have to climb down from our revolving horses and look at reality if we are to force government agencies, presumably designed to protect us and care for our best interests, to finally be accountable.

Until the full extent of what has actually happened to us in the Hanford area and in many other parts of the country is finally admitted and examined, all nuclear facilities should halt production. It is critical that political expediency not play a part in this issue, for if we can't make our world safe we won't have to fear being destroyed by the Soviets or anyone else. We'll destroy ourselves, and our cemeteries will be "hot" for centuries.

NOTES

1. Schumacher, Eloise, "Radioactive release is remembered in Fremont exhibit," *Seattle Times*, December 3, 1989, p. B-1.
2. Bingman, Teresa, "Cancer rate alarms health officials," *East Washingtonian*, January 2, 1986.
3. Cecil, Nelta, "Water supply scheduled for cancer testing," *East Washingtonian*, February 5, 1986.
4. Veseth, Roger, "Radioactive Fallout Provides Estimator for Soil Erosion," *Growers Guide*, May/June, 1990, pp. A12-A15.

The Legacy

KAREN HOPKINS
as told to Judith Brady

"**B**ut, Your Honor," I told the judge as tears streamed down my face, "I'm a single mother with two kids."

The judge wasn't impressed. Then I blurted, "And I've got cancer."

"Do you have any proof that you have cancer?" he asked, unmoved by my sobbing.

"No," I said. "I didn't think I would have to come here today with anything like that."

The judge was clearly irritated. "You stand before me with $400 worth of warrants for outstanding traffic tickets and no proof of the cancer you claim. I will have to sentence you to $400 bail and to 100 hours of community service."

I couldn't believe he would do this to me. He gave me by far the most severe penalty of any he had meted out that morning, and he even put me on parking ticket probation so that if I got another parking ticket I could go to jail. That judge didn't know it, but he gave me a lot more than a stern punishment for outstanding traffic tickets. For me his sentence was also the beginning of a very different understanding of my cancer and a very different conception of my world.

I work for the city police in the criminal investigation department. When the city switched health plans for city workers, my doctor noticed that my records showed a nodule on my thyroid gland, a lump I had discovered years ago. The doctor under my old plan did a needle biopsy, and he told me that everything was okay since such nodules were pretty common, especially in people who had had many X-rays. The new doctor thought he should check it out, however, so he had called me in to have another routine needle biopsy. One morning, six months prior to my court appearance, the new doctor called me at work. "I'm sorry to tell you," he said, "but I just got the pathology reports, and your test was positive; you have malignant cancer . . ."

I never even heard the rest of what he said. I dropped the telephone and began crying uncontrollably. My lieutenant offered to drive me to the doctor's office. He dropped me off, and I went into the doctor's waiting room, still crying. The doctor told me that it was rare for a needle biopsy to show such unmistakably malignant cells; usually a biopsy just indicated that further tests should be made. But my case was clear, and he wanted me to see a surgeon right away. I knew I was going to die.

I went across the street to see a surgeon, who told me all the risks and then set up a surgery date for the following Friday—the day on which I was going to start a week of vacation with my kids. I went back to work, arranged to have the time off, and then I called my kids and told them the vacation was cancelled. I also told my kids, I remember, that it was okay to be mad at me; I remembered how I felt when my grandfather died and I couldn't go to a dance.

Then I started getting ready for the ordeal ahead. My affairs were in order. I had made a will. I felt that my oldest boy could handle whatever happened and take care of his younger brother. I was prepared to die.

The surgery went well. They removed nearly all the gland and put me on thyroid supplements. I was supposed to stay home for six weeks, but in three weeks I felt I had to go back to work because I needed to be around people. So back I went, with my neck swathed in white bandages.

Parking near my workplace had always been a problem. There were meters everywhere, so if you didn't remember to move your car or feed the meter, you would get a ticket. I remember thinking, when I returned to work with my bandages, that it was okay if I got a parking ticket. I wasn't going to live out the year anyway. So, I thought, I might as well make myself as comfortable as possible until I die. I parked at the meters every day and paid no attention to the tickets.

With the same nonchalant attitude, I took my son on a shopping spree and bought a brand new television. Then I bought some new stereo equipment. I pretty quickly went through my savings. While I was busy consoling myself by spending, I was also accumulating more parking tickets.

Six months went by, and I was still alive. The bills started coming in, and the tickets had gone into warrants. I had to set a date to appear before the traffic commissioner. When I tearfully announced to the judge that I had cancer, I was trying to tell him that collecting traffic tickets was not my usual way of doing things. Normally I am a very responsible person. I pay my bills.

I had never done anything like this before, but I was in this fix now because I was sure I was going to die. Instead of getting sympathy, I just made the judge angry. I paid my fine, and then had to face the 100 hours of community service.

I went to an agency which tries to match a person's skills to the needs of an approved non-profit organization through which I could work off my 100 hours. I had a hard time trying to figure out what my skills were. I could dust for fingerprints and collect blood from crime scenes, but those didn't seem like appropriate skills for non-profit organizations. I had, however, learned to type in high school. I was given the telephone number of an agency which needed typing help. The address was that of a house in a very nice neighborhood, and the woman who ran the agency said she could take me on my schedule.

I drove to the house, and Dorothy Legaretta, the woman with whom I had spoken, greeted me and took me to her office on the third floor of the house. She was very pleasant and friendly with me. She was an older woman who had had ten children. She had just recently gotten her Ph.D., and she had written a book. I was quite impressed; not many women could boast of such accomplishments. I began typing labels for her, and then after a while I asked her what this organization was for which I was doing all this typing.

She told me that her organization, the National Association of Radiation Survivors (NARS), was locating and collecting data on people who had been exposed to radiation, principally servicemen who had taken part in Operation Crossroads in 1946, in which the United States tested the impact of nuclear weapons by dropping a bomb over the Marshall Islands. I am a political conservative, and I was quite taken aback when she told me what that organization was doing. Oh, God, I thought, I've gotten myself into a liberal house . . . these people are always so damn gung-ho . . . I continued to type the letters which Dorothy dictated, but I had no interest at all in what she was saying.

By my third visit to the NARS office I was typing a lot of the statistics that Dorothy had been gathering about people who were sick from radiation damage. Then Dorothy began asking me questions about why I had to do 100 hours of community service. She knew I was a real conservative, and she knew that I had once worked for the FBI. It occurred to me later that she might be thinking that I was some sort of a plant. I told her about my parking tickets and about my cancer surgery.

"What kind of cancer did you have?" she asked.

"Thyroid," I answered.

She told me that she had had thyroid surgery, too, and that was why she was doing the work she was doing. She had been carelessly exposed to excessive radiation in 1944 when she worked as a young laboratory technician at the Crocker Radiation Lab which led research in the Manhattan Project, which developed and produced the atomic bomb. I brushed that information aside, though in the course of our conversation I told her that my youngest son had been born deaf. I had been reading about a lot of cases like my son in the statistical charts I was typing.

Dorothy told me that one of her ten children, a son, had died of leukemia. Then she asked me if my father had been in the service. It was true that my father had been in the service, but most fathers of people my age had been in the service.

"Yes," I answered her, "he was in the Navy."

"What year?" she asked.

"He started in 1943," I said, "and he was a twenty-year vet."

"Did he ever talk about what he did in the service?"

I told her no, that he was a very quiet person who didn't talk much about anything, but I knew he had been out on ships.

Dorothy handed me a list of ships and asked me if he had been on any of them. I said I wouldn't know. She asked if I could find out from him. He was dead, I told her.

"When did he die?" she asked. I told her years ago, but I couldn't remember exactly.

"What did he die of?" she wanted to know.

I told her that he had died of some rare form of esophageal cancer.

"Oh," she said. "Well, could your mom give you the information?"

No, I told her; my mother was also dead.

"When did she die?" Dorothy asked.

I remember when my mother died because my son had just been born. When Dorothy asked me what my mother had died of, I answered that my mother had died very quickly at the age of forty-four from acute leukemia.

Dorothy just looked at me. Her mouth dropped open a bit. "Do you know," she quietly asked me, "that your father had probably been exposed to radiation?"

When I asked her what she meant, she showed me a chart she had compiled representing the illnesses of men who had been exposed to radiation in the Pacific during the Marshall Islands testing of atom bombs in 1946. A lot of those people had died and more were still dying from various cancers. The chart illustrated when the illnesses had shown up, what had happened with the children of those men, and even what had happened with their grandchildren—more cancers and more genetic disorders.

She asked me more questions. She asked if there were migraine headaches in my family. I told her that I had a brother and a sister, both of whom suffered from migraine headaches. My oldest boy also had migraine headaches. She knew my youngest son had been born deaf. I didn't understand how my mother's leukemia could be connected to any possible radiation exposure to my father, but Dorothy said that a lot of the wives of men who had been exposed to radiation also developed cancers, probably because the wives had done the laundry of the men who came home wearing clothes covered with radioactive dust. It would take years for the cancers to develop, of course. And my mother's leukemia developed almost exactly twenty years after my father had been stationed at Hunters Point, a Navy shipyard in San Francisco, where the target ships from Operation Crossroads in the Bikini atoll of the Marshall Islands had been taken.

What Dorothy showed me about my own cancer, my sons' physical difficulties, and the deaths of my parents ran counter to everything I had understood and taken for granted. My father had taught me that whatever our government did was for our greatest good, and that it was right to support the government and wrong to fight it. My father believed in what he was doing; he had joined the Navy when he was sixteen. He even lied about his age and forged papers so that he could go to war for his country. He was very proud of what he had done, and it was clear that he was prepared to die for his country. He would never have said anything against the United States. When my father died he might have known that his cancer was a result of radiation exposure. I don't know. But even if he did know, he never said anything against the government.

I grew up being taught that it is wrong to lie and cheat, and it is also wrong to be disloyal to your country. I believed that. I went to work for the FBI when I was seventeen years old. I found out that the FBI was involved in illegal activities, but I believed that the FBI was justified because they were fighting an even greater evil. I didn't really have opinions of my own. I believed in whatever the Bureau believed, and I never did have a private opinion which opposed the views of the Bureau. Even if I had, I would never have said anything about it.

Yet I believed Dorothy. It was eerie that I didn't have to tell Dorothy anything; she told me about my life before I told her. As she questioned me about my past and about my parents, she described events in my life to me even before I had mentioned them. She had collected data about hundreds of people whose stories sounded a lot like mine. I began to find myself believing what those people I had thought of as "screaming liberals" had been saying about nuclear testing.

And I felt that Dorothy really cared. She was very excited about the work she was doing, but I could also see that she cared about me because of my cancer and because of what had happened to my parents and my son. When I had finished my 100 hours of community service, I continued to work with Dorothy as a volunteer. Dorothy and NARS had a big effect on me. I was impressed that NARS managed to operate so well on a shoestring and that they had so many volunteers. And I was moved by Dorothy's dedication. Whenever I went to a fund-raising educational event for NARS with Dorothy, she was the first one to write out a check to her own organization.

After Dorothy's death in a car accident last year I stopped working with NARS. Her death took a lot of energy out of the organization, and for me the organization has changed.

I think, too, that I stay away from NARS because of my fear. I don't want to look too closely at the reality of how many people in this country are affected by these cancers that relate to the Bikini Island bomb testing, the testing of the bombs that the government said they "weren't going to use" but that were going to "make us a strong nation." Those tests are still being repeated many times a year at the Nevada Test Site. Why, I wonder. Who wants to collect results from these tests? We already know that radiation poisoning is not a good thing. I had a cousin who lived in Beatty, Nevada, the nearest town to the Nevada Test Site, during those early tests, and she died of leukemia at the age of twenty. Her name was Charlotte. I never did say anything to my aunt and uncle about my suspicions. Why does the government have to keep on, year after year, spreading more and more of that poison?

All that ground is polluted and it doesn't go away.

It wasn't until I heard about this anthology that I started looking for my father's records. Until then I didn't want to know exactly where he had been; I didn't think I could handle the truth even though I now believe that my thyroid cancer is linked to his exposure to radiation. He might have been in the South Pacific. I did find out that he had been in Hunters Point before I was born in 1949, where all the target ships from Operation Crossroads were brought. There they tried to clean up those ships, make them no longer radioactive. They tried all sorts of things. Even cornstarch. They thought that cornstarch would soak up the radiation.

Nothing worked, of course. Eventually, they sold some of the hot ships to other countries as scrap metal. Others they towed out to the Pacific Ocean and sank. Some of those hot ships were sunk in the paths of migratory fish which are still caught and sold to people as food. Then they sank some of those radioactive ships right here in our San Francisco Bay.

That radioactivity will last for thousands of years; there is nothing we can do to fix it. All we can do is stop adding to it. Education is the key, I think; people in this country need to be educated. There are a lot of people out there who are like me, who grew up believing in our country, right or wrong. My brother and sister, for instance, still don't want to hear about our father, even though they both have migraine headaches.

I have pretty much come to accept that I might die of this cancer. My fear is about what will happen with my children. And I think about the children of my brother; his daughters are both very young yet and seem to be perfectly normal and healthy, but the possibility that something might appear in one of them is too strong. My oldest son will probably be the first one to produce the next generation, and I worry about that, too.

Our government needs to be doing education about radiation exposure, and we need to be doing research on other forms of producing energy. But first we need to acknowledge what has already happened so that we can deal with what has already been done to so many people.

An American Hibakusha

MILLIE SMITH

In 1945 the U.S. government dropped an atomic bomb on Hiroshima, Japan and then another one on Nagasaki. The Japanese have a name for their citizens who lived through the bombings but who suffered from the radiation exposure. The victims of the atomic bomb, their children and their children's children are called Hibakusha.

While the bomb which destroyed Nagasaki was being secretly produced at the Hanford Nuclear Power Plant in Washington, that same nuclear plant was also silently and secretly releasing invisible radioactive particles into its own community, a practice which continued for many years. I was born in 1947 and raised in Pasco, Washington, several miles downstream from the Hanford Nuclear Plant. I am an American Hibakusha.

In 1986 I learned the truth about Hanford, and shortly before Christmas of that year my metastasized thyroid cancer was discovered. The doctors said I could have had it for twenty years. In horrified disbelief I sought a second opinion, and that doctor told me that I probably would not last for two more years and that immediate surgery was my only hope.

No matter how often one thinks about death, nothing can prepare you for actually being confronted by it. As I walked out of the doctor's office, everything in the world seemed changed. Time had slowed. In need of comfort and shelter, I thought of the man with whom I was involved. I was confident that his love for me would help me bear this sudden awful burden. But that trust was shattered when on Christmas Eve I told him what had happened to me, and he walked out. Then the devastating reality of my illness really hit me. I would have to face it alone.

Rapidly I grew weaker and my voice more hoarse. I was urged not to delay surgery any longer, but fear held me back. There was too much I didn't know. Desperately I sought information about the thyroid gland, cancer, and the effects of radiation.

Every book I read told me that the most common cause of thyroid cancer was from exposure to radiation, and that those who were exposed as children were the most seriously affected.

Besides being carried in the air, radioactive iodine accumulates in various foods and in milk, concentrating in the thyroid after consumption. The thyroid regulates metabolism, and any malfunction can cause serious health problems which can affect other organs of the body. In fact, I learned that even normal doses of pain medication or barbiturates given to someone with severe undetected hypothyroidism can be fatal.

Thyroid surgery is very delicate, and there are differences of opinion regarding the best procedure. Possible complications from the surgery include paralysis of the vocal cords and tracheostomy. I did not want to have a tracheostomy. I did not want to lose my thyroid. I did not want to die. I sent for my medical report and learned that my jugular vein was also involved, and in fact was barely working. No one could tell me what that meant, either. Terrified though I was, I finally agreed to have the surgery. Later I learned that my surgery was considered nearly miraculous. The cancer had spread throughout my neck and upper chest, and there were tumors on my laryngeal nerve, which also had to be removed.

It took me many months to recover. I lay in my bed, longing for the trees, the ocean, the sun. Frustrating as it was for me to be so incapacitated, the experience of my convalescence from surgery was even harder on my thirteen-year-old daughter, who had to bear the full burden of caring for me. I wasn't able then to appreciate what she must have been feeling, fearing that she might lose me. She seemed afraid to be too close.

As my strength returned, friends brought me books so that I could continue my research on radiation. As I read and reflected back on my own life, pieces of the puzzle began to fall into place. All of my other physical problems as well as the thyroid cancer could have been results of radiation exposure. The strange, unexplained disabilities with which I had struggled fit the profile of people who had been exposed to radiation as children.[1] Even the changes in my mental abilities as a teenager fit the picture. I wondered about other people from the Tri-Cities area, and I began remembering the childhood friends of mine who had died of cancer while still in their youth. I remembered, too, the many cancer deaths of aunts and cousins in my own family, as well as the deaths of family friends.

During this time, I met Tom Bailie, a farmer near Hanford. He told me that on his land, adjacent to the Hanford Reservation, twenty-four out of twenty-eight families were seriously affected by thyroid disorders, cancers, and serious birth defects.[2,3]

When a recurrence of the malignant tumor was detected in my neck, I feared the radioactive iodine treatment prescribed by my doctors as much as I feared the spreading cancer. It didn't seem reasonable that the radioactive iodine which had caused my cancer could also be a cure. I would have to be in isolation for four days, with food and water slipped under the door. My turmoil increased when I learned that the proposed radiation treatment also posed the risk of leukemia and further damage to my reproductive organs.

My fear of the cancer spreading to my trachea or my lungs finally grew to be greater than my fear of the treatment. I had the radiation, but only in doses small enough that I could avoid isolation. My tumor was destroyed, as well as what was left of my thyroid. And no matter what the doctors say, I am just not the same with my thyroid gone.

In the summer of 1988 I met a group of Japanese people who had come to Hanford on a peace mission. As we floated silently down the Columbia River, past the nuclear plant which had not only destroyed their country but our lives in the Hanford area as well, a powerful bond developed between us. I felt a flourishing connection to those people who had also been damaged by my government. The unity I felt with them aided my healing process.

In August of that year I made a visit to Japan with fellow downwinder Tom Bailie. It was there that I first spoke out about my life as a survivor of radiation exposure, and it was in Japan that I learned how important it is to tell our stories as witnesses to what happened at Hanford. People in Japan who had refused before to even speak to Americans came to talk to Tom and me. My life at home had been years of pain, poverty and denial. In Japan I found compassion, understanding, and recognition as Hibakusha. Doctors there were surprised that my health history was identical to their Hibakusha patients—the thyroid cancer, birth defects, susceptibility to infections and illness, lethargy, weakness, dizziness, nausea and vomiting, heavy nosebleeds, septicemia, inability to work or handle stress, environmental illness. As I learned about the genetic effects from radiation on future generations, I not only feared for my daughter, but for all the future children of the world.

I was especially moved by Hiroshima, a city which withstood one of the worse forms of destruction known to mankind and arose out of its ashes to become a city of peace. I placed a wreath in atonement at one memorial, and I felt as though I had come home. People from all over the world had visited this memorial, coming in peace, love and reverence. Together, the Japanese and the American Hibakusha set lighted lanterns afloat down the river out to sea to honor souls lost to the bomb which had destroyed us both.

Forty years after the war, the Hibakusha all over Japan are still ill. And still some of what they suffer evades medical understanding. Medical care is free for most of the survivors, and there are several hospitals and treatment centers especially for atomic bomb victims. But there is also social discrimination against bomb victims. Others do not want to marry them for fear of giving birth to children who will have genetic defects. There have been many suicides by bomb victims who felt helpless and misunderstood while battling strange ailments which baffled both doctors and patients alike.

When I returned to the United States, I began to write and speak out whenever I could, feeling driven despite my poor health, never forgetting my experiences in Japan. I completed a health survey on former high school classmates, and I learned of more cancer deaths and more multiple health problems. Hundreds of stories emerge from other downwinders and from people who used to work at the Hanford plant. More secret documents came to light, confirming that even higher amounts of radiation than we thought had been released and substantiating the increased health risks.

But it isn't just Hanford. Disaster reports about nuclear power plants across the country are in the news. It is impossible to know how many people have been unknowingly damaged. It is impossible even to know if the contaminated land and water can ever be cleaned from the vast quantities of radioactive waste.

If my story could make a difference, it would be worth everything I have endured. I am just one of thousands affected by the silent Hanford tragedy and one of at least a million Americans estimated by the National Association of Radiation Survivors who have been exposed to harmful amounts of radiation. What legacy do we leave to our children? The Japanese Hibakusha and we downwinders—the American Hibakusha—have been exposed to the wind of death. It is my hope that future generations will be spared the horrors so many have endured as victims of nuclear proliferation.

NOTES

1. Sternglass, Ernest, *Secret Fallout*, McGraw Hill, Hightstown, NJ, 1972.
2. Personal conversation with Tom Bailie, November, 1987.
3. "Searching for Atomic Bomb Victims," *New York Times*, October 17, 1988, p. 1.

III. Surviving the Cure: Dealing with the Medical Profession

Pay on the Way Out

JUNE BEISCH

It is the policy of this
hospital to let you know
the alternative treatments, and although
you are free to choose, I feel I must
advise you against the choice you have made
I feel it would be in your best
interests to remove the whole breast
but since you refuse

I must warn you

I feel I should tell you
I can't promise you a cure
You may regret it I can't be sure
Most women I know will not take that risk
And all of the cure rates are still not in

You may end up paying for it
on the way out. Take a little time
to think about it.

Stop at the desk on your way out please
Goodbye, good luck
pay on the way out.

Choices: Personal Reflections on the Politics of Cancer

SIMI LITVAK

Following a routine mammogram I was told that a suspicious lump had been found in my breast. This discovery was the beginning of an experience which made it clear to me that in our country the class background of patients determines the sort of medical treatment we will receive, and it became further clear to me that politics and economics—not our health or lack of it—determine the choices we will have.

Once cancer is suspected, patients are faced with having to make a series of complex decisions in a very short time. We may have to agree to some type of diagnostic procedure. If cancer is confirmed, we may also have to choose between several alternative surgical procedures, and then we may have to decide whether or not we will agree to a recommendation of chemotherapy and/or radiation. These judgments must be made quickly, and we have to gather as much information as possible in order to make them, all the while contending with the shock of finding out that we have cancer.

When breast cancer is the issue, the typical strictly hierarchical relationship between the woman cancer patient and her physician has given way partially to the appearance of a more egalitarian relationship. During the past several decades, women have demanded a greater say in what happens to our bodies. In many states physicians are obliged by law to advise a breast cancer patient of all her possible options, and doctors are attempting to avoid liability by requiring patients to participate more in deciding treatment preferences. Yet, even though we women are given more latitude in making choices, we are not automatically armed with the information necessary to exercise that hard-won right to some self-determination.

How we deal with the pressure of decision-making is not totally a matter of personal psychology. Rather, our ability to function when faced with choices is highly dependent upon how much help we can get and how much information is made available to us. It is also dependent on our access to expert medical advice and treatment. In the United States, that access to help and expertise appears to depend largely upon our class position.

I am an occupational therapist with a Ph.D. At every point in my own cancer journey I was acutely aware of how my educational background, employment status as a researcher with flexible work hours, Health Maintenance Organization (HMO) benefits, state disability insurance, ability to afford private psychotherapy, and residence in a large, progressive urban area with very developed women's and alternative health resources and information centers were all factors which made it possible for me to get information. In fact, even my ability to read was a significant advantage. Nearly a third of the adult population in the United States is functionally illiterate.[1] Many other people do not read English. Neither the illiterate population nor non-English readers would be readily able to use the volumes of medical pamphlets, women's movement resources, and alternative health literature which were essential to me in sorting through the numerous baffling choices I faced.

Because I have experience in the medical profession and because I had knowledge of and access to information and resources developed through the women's movement, I knew I had to inform myself about the medical procedure before I even saw a surgeon for a biopsy, and I knew how to go about getting that information. I knew about the existence of a national cancer hotline, and I called it. The counselor who answered my call was extremely helpful and sent me loads of information pertaining to the diagnostic phase of cancer treatment.

Thanks to the details I got through the hotline, I knew enough to reject my first HMO-assigned surgeon. He wanted me to sign a consent form for a biopsy without even explaining what was on the form. The second surgeon was much more communicative, and the biopsy went smoothly. The pathologist examined the tissue sample and found cancer.

I was told that I needed more surgery to ensure that all the cancerous tissue was removed and to determine if the cancer cells had spread to the lymph nodes under my arm. I could choose a procedure which removed more tissue around the area where the lump had been before the biopsy by having a lumpectomy, which would preserve my breast and which would be followed by radiation. Or I could choose the surgical removal of my breast in a mastectomy. My HMO doctor gave me a handout comparing the two procedures, said he would be available for questions, and sent me home. I had to make this very tough decision in one week because my surgeon was going out of town and wanted to allow time for post-operative follow-up.

Through the women's movement press I had heard about the Women's Cancer Resource Center. Over the weekend I tracked them down, and they put me in touch with one woman who had had a lumpectomy and with another woman who had had a mastectomy. This personal contact with firsthand experience was very important to me. The woman with a mastectomy sent me a dramatic poster of an inspirational poem illustrated with a photograph of a joyful woman whose arms were outstretched and her mastectomy scar tattooed with grape vines.[2] The poster with the poem became a powerful symbol of recovery for me. My lover hung twelve copies all around my hospital room.

Not all offerings from my friends, however, were as supportive as the poster. While I was going through the process of trying to make my treatment determination, some well-meaning friends gave me an audiotape made by Louise Hay, a New Age self-proclaimed healer. I have heard from other women that they, too, received New Age books and tapes from well-meaning friends as soon as the word was out that they had cancer. I listened to the Hay tape.

The essence of the Hay message was that I caused myself to have cancer because I had accumulated regrets and resentment in my past and present lives. I thought of the world I know and of the hundreds of thousands of people who get cancer every year. Did the residents of Love Canal, whose homes were built over a toxic waste dump, cause their own cancers? Did the uranium miners in New Mexico and those in Colorado, whose town was built on uranium pilings, cause their own cancers from unresolved resentments? Do the children of farmworkers in the pesticide-drenched agricultural fields who develop leukemia cause that cancer to invade their bodies?

Appalled, I turned my back on New Age views, and focused on the search for more surgery information. The Cancer Information Center sent excellent literature, and the counselor told me that two months earlier (June, 1988) the National Cancer Institute (NCI) sent a letter to all cancer treatment facilities recommending chemotherapy for all women diagnosed with breast cancer regardless of lymph node involvement;[3] before this new approach, women without lymph node involvement did not routinely receive chemotherapy. I tried to discuss this new approach with my surgeon, but he put me off by saying that such a question should be saved for the post-operative phase. I didn't agree; I wanted to understand the background of this new approach so I could make an informed decision about a lumpectomy with radiation as opposed to a mastectomy, because if I chose the lumpectomy, I might be exposing myself to both radiation and chemotherapy. So I asked for a referral to the radiologist to hear the pros and cons of lumpectomy with radiation and how that would be done if I also had chemotherapy.

Finally, I felt I had gathered all the information I could. As I thought about what I had learned, I realized that with a relatively small tumor like mine there really was no obvious choice between mastectomy and lumpectomy. There are advantages and disadvantages to both. In the end, the decision would rest on personal preferences. I had to decide how I felt about not having one breast, how I felt about having radiation, and how I felt about chemotherapy. Going to a therapist helped me make my choice, but I had to keep repeating to myself that whatever I chose, that choice would be the right one.

I decided to have a mastectomy because I did not want more radiation. Some years earlier I had been diagnosed with thyroid cancer which required the removal of half my thyroid gland. Thyroid cancer is associated with radiation exposure, and until I was an adult I lived sixteen miles from Rocky Flats in Colorado where a plutonium spill occurred in the mid-fifties, approximately eighteen years before my thyroid cancer was discovered. It was not until very recently, however, that I learned about exposure to ionizing radiation also being a major factor in breast cancer.

Once I had made the decision, I prepared for the operation. Recovery from the mastectomy went well. I got some help from the surgeon, the nurses, and an American Cancer Society volunteer, but my knowledge of muscles from working as an occupational therapist was very important in retaining full motion in my arm. And I could take enough time from work for convalescence because I received disability payments from the state of California, a benefit which is not available in every state and not available to all workers in any state.

My next decision concerned chemotherapy. I had some understandable reservations about chemotherapy; I knew several people who had received it and suffered its side effects. So I went to PlaneTree, a medical library for non-medical people, but there was very little on file about adjuvant chemotherapy for breast cancer. I couldn't find the studies on which the new guidelines from the National Cancer Institute were based; instead, there seemed to be a lot of controversy regarding the efficacy of adjuvant chemotherapy. The Women's Cancer Resource Center came to my aid again. They suggested that I get a second opinion and recommended a pathologist at one of San Francisco's leading hospitals who specializes in breast cancer. My HMO would not pay for me to see someone outside the HMO system, but this was a big decision and I needed excellent advice. I am luckier than many cancer patients; even though I had to make sacrifices, I could come up with the money to pay for it.

The pathologist examined the slides from my HMO laboratory and concluded that I had a totally different cancer type from what the HMO pathologists had determined. The difference between the two opinions was crucial. The HMO pathologist said I had a type of cancer that is fast growing and has a high possibility of returning or spreading. The pathologist at the other hospital said that my slides indicated another type of cancer, atypical medullary carcinoma. Only one definitive study had ever been done on medullary and atypical medullary carcinoma because they were so rare that it was difficult to find enough people to study. That one study showed, however, that medullary cancer was much less likely to recur, even without chemotherapy.[4, 5]

My HMO oncologist, when he had read the two conflicting pathology reports, told me that pathologists were notorious for having contradictory opinions, and in any event, he concluded, people with medullary cancer were probably included in the NCI studies and thus the findings regarding adjuvant chemotherapy applied to them as well. His reasoning made no sense to me; possibly one or two people with medullary carcinoma could not be statistically significant. I asked that the slides be re-examined by the HMO pathologists. One agreed with the outside pathologist, and four upheld the first diagnosis. I was caught between two teams of doctors.

I'm not a pathologist. But I can understand the research, and I was not convinced that chemotherapy would appreciably increase my chances for survival. I spoke again to the outside pathologist;

he went through the research study with me and answered all my questions, but I was still uncertain about what to do. He explained to me that I was caught between a community hospital (the HMO) which treated all types of breast cancer based on the same protocol and a research center specializing in breast cancer which separates women into groups based on their type of breast cancer and follows them over a long period of time in order to differentiate between the courses of their diseases and distinctive treatments required. That made sense.

He then suggested that I get a third opinion from another pathologist who specialized in breast cancer. I chose one of the two names he gave me, and he sent the slides to that pathologist. The third opinion came back with even better news than the second! This specialist determined that I had medullary carcinoma, the survival rates for which are even higher than for atypical medullary carcinoma. Now I was able to make my decision. I said no to chemotherapy.

My experience with cancer is not over yet, however. I still receive more New Age literature from well-meaning friends with more subtle messages about my own culpability in my disease. I think that people like Bernie Siegel,[6] the Simontons,[7] and Norman Cousins,[8] who maintain that our attitudes and behavior both determine our illness and are of primary importance in our healing, do have a point. Our attitudes probably do influence how we react to disease and trauma. Two people can have identical diagnoses and one will choose to fight like hell while the other may just give in. But even those who choose to fight back by making significant behavioral, lifestyle, and attitudinal changes do so within the limits of their pre-existing health status, the disease process, and the class-determined array of choices available to them.

Furthermore, the whole theory of a "cancer personality" is based on very poor science. The Simontons, who developed the theory, based it upon their observations of cancer patients who came to their office, some of whom were quite distressed. But people with cancer are not the only ones in our society who are depressed, resentful, and filled with regret. We live in a highly competitive, alienating society which breeds those feelings. So far, attempts to conclusively prove the reality of a cancer personality theory have failed, though unfortunately this failure has not yet trickled down to all the producers of cancer self-cure books.

In the meantime, the sellers of self-blame (or "responsibility") do people with cancer psychological harm at the very time when we need to marshal all our psychic strength to deal with the cancer. Even worse, perhaps, is that assigning the cause for cancer to oneself has deflected people from recognizing and fighting against the ultimate cause of cancer: environmental pollution and the lack of adequate health care to combat it.

As people in my social and family circles learned that I had cancer, individuals began approaching me with their cancer stories. Several people asked for information to help them support friends with cancer. Two of my first cousins called for advice and resource references when their cancers were diagnosed. One eventually died of cancer, as did my lover's mother, less than a year after I was diagnosed.

I began to realize how many people either have cancer themselves or have experienced it with friends, co-workers and families. The numbers of people facing cancer are staggering. More women, for instance, die of breast cancer alone every year than do all the people who have AIDS.

People who are poor suffer the highest rates of cancer.[9] And since poverty in our society coincides with race and ethnicity, a disproportionate number of people of color in the United States have cancer, along with all the other ills of poverty. This reality is no surprise when one considers that 37 million working Americans have no health insurance at all because they work for employers who do not provide insurance or because they have health conditions which make them ineligible for health insurance. Many more millions of people in this country have inadequate insurance, which does not cover preventive measures such as periodic mammograms or second opinions. When I think about the advice I sought at every step of my treatment and how it influenced the course of my treatment, I cannot help but realize how important my insurance and my ability to pay for second and third opinions were.

As my awareness of the enormity of the cancer epidemic has grown, so has my anger. Our economic system has created a multi-tiered medical system in which class and race are dominant determinants of the advice, treatment, and potential for survival one can expect. For several decades scientists have noted the link between environmental chemical and nuclear pollution and the rising incidence of cancer. Yet the bulk of research on cancer in the United States is aimed at cure, not prevention.[10] It seems to me that there are two principal reasons for this apparent lack of logic. First, true prevention would compel checking the growth of industrial pollution and would therefore require major production changes. Secondly, research into prevention would not yield a drug or technological "cure" which would reap some company enormous profits.

It is only now that all levels of our class-stratified society are impacted by the cancer epidemic—not just working people who are forced to live and work close to the sources of pollution—that environmental issues are being debated as a part of national and international policy. The survival of the human race is at stake.

NOTES

1. Kozol, Jonathan, "A Third of the Nation Cannot Read These Words," *The Shape of This Century*, Diana W. Rigen and Susan S. Waugh, eds., Harcourt Brace Jovanovich, Orlando, Florida, 1990, p. 529.
2. Metzger, Deena, "Tree," Wingbow Press, San Francisco.
3. Zoler, M. L., "Breast Cancer Alert Draws Rapid Fire from Oncologists," *Medical World News*, June 27, 1988, p. 22.
4. Ridolfi, R.L., P.O. Rosen, et al., "Medullary Carcinoma of the Breast: A Clinicopathologic Study with 10 Year Follow-up," *Cancer* 40 (40):1365-1385, 1977.
5. Rapin, V., et al., "Medullary Breast Carcinoma: A Reevaluation of 95 Cases of Breast Cancer with Inflammatory Stroma," *Cancer* 61 (10):2503-2510, 1988.
6. Siegel, B., *Love, Medicine and Miracles: Lessons Learned about Self-Healing From a Surgeon's Experience with Exceptional Patients*, Harper and Row, New York, 1989.
7. Simonton, O.C., S. Simonton, et al., *Getting Well Again*, Bantam Books, New York, 1980.
8. Cousins, N., *Anatomy of an Illness as Perceived by the Patient*, Bantam Books, New York, 1981.
9. Cimons, Marlene, "Poor more likely to die needlessly of cancer, National Study finds," *Oakland Tribune*, July 18, 1989. From a study released July 17, 1989 by the American Cancer Society.
10. Epstein, S. S., *The Politics of Cancer*, Anchor Books, Garden City, New York, 1979.

The Generic Oncologist

HELENE DAVIS

"Why are you here?" is the first question he asks me. Why am I here? Over his desk, facing his patients, are photographs of his entire family: wife, children, even a dog. Why are they there? Are they there to reassure me that there are families, that I might get one? Are they there to reassure him that he won't catch my sadness, my fear? Are they a Greek chorus saying, "Cancer, cancer. Step up and say the word that explains why you are here"?

But I know better, and I do not want to say the word that changes life into something else. I sit on my uncomfortable chair, flanked by two good friends, and say it: "I am here for chemotherapy." And the wife and the children and the dog look on at the doctor and me. "Are there any questions?" he asks after giving me heart-stopping statistics. This is serious business, the statistics say.

I am speechless for the first time I can remember. My friends ask articulate questions, notebooks in hand. I am told I will remember little of this interview. I inch into my body and a world where none of this is happening. I hear little, say little, but my friends write everything down. "How long do I have?" I ask silently, not wanting to know. I hear him say, "You are going to lose your hair." I say, "I lost my breast, now I am going to lose my hair." "Your hair grows back," he says.

Skeletons

BARBARA HOFFMAN

In the cold summer room
we wait
for the iodine
to irradiate our bones
I'm subject #2301
in this free study
on bone pain
in breast cancer patients

you, subject #2302
cancer six years ago
you'd been feeling good
but, lately, lately
you've dropped some weight
and your jawbone hurts

Dr. Research leads us
down barren halls
to the bone scan room
I stand on the metal half-moon
my back against the giant circle
think of the old silent movies
with the woman strapped
to a wheel spinning
until the hero rushes in

"Don't move," he says
as the geiger counter clicks
my skeleton in neon yellow
on his computer screen
he points at my glowing frame
his face lit up by my bones

after the test
#2302, you say
goodbye   goodluck
the skin on your nose
falls away
leaving a fine straight bone
your eye sockets deepen
your face disintegrates
your skeleton unfolds

A Letter to My Doctor

CINDY WINSLOW

To My Doctor:

It is with reluctance that I write this letter to you, though I think such a letter could be written to many physicians in this country by many patients. We are all caught in a system which makes both giving and receiving quality health care nearly impossible.

It does seem, however, that patients—not physicians—are paying the heaviest price for a health care system which simply does not work. In terms of my particular relationship with you, it is clear to me now that you can no longer be my primary care physician. Please send my records to the physician who will take your place and who my insurance company promises will be accessible.

Before any more time passes, I want to explain myself more fully than I could in the heat of our last accidental encounter in the hospital cafeteria. I hope that this letter will clarify the issues and leave us both with more peace of mind or at least a clearer understanding of the situation in which we both find ourselves. It is painful for me to look back upon the history of my connection with your office, but I think you need to know how I see it.

In January, 1988, I called your office upon the recommendation of an acquaintance who spoke highly of you. I have never before had the need to see a physician regularly because I never had any serious health problems. When I did need to see a doctor for an annual Pap smear, checkup, or the occasional flu, I went to whomever my insurance company recommended.

But I knew that something was really wrong with my body the day I called your office. In the preceding four months I had gained thirty pounds, my skin was consistently bad, my stools were irregular, I lacked energy, and I couldn't hold my urine. I was informed by your office that I had to wait three months for an appointment. I had already waited months for my employer's health insurance to become effective. But even though I felt miserable, no particular symptom seemed acute, so I patiently waited for three months to see you.

When my April appointment date finally arrived, I read to you my list of symptoms, a list I had carefully prepared so I could give you all the information you might need. You addressed each of the symptoms as an isolated complaint. My Pap smear and pelvic examination results were negative. I was given pills to compensate for a hypo-active thyroid and more pills to kill an intestinal parasite. You suggested that my incontinence was due to the failing muscle tone which accompanies aging. I was a bit puzzled by the news about aging; I am only thirty-six and have always been athletic. In response to my request for nutritional advice, you tossed me a photocopy of a diet as I was on my way out the door and suggested that I lose five pounds before my next visit in three weeks to check on the thyroid medication. But when the thyroid lab tests proved the current dosage was correct, your nurse cancelled my follow-up appointment to check my weight. So I set out on my own course of daily aerobics and organized weight loss, and I assumed I would see you in another year for a routine Pap smear.

A few months later, twenty pounds lighter and with firm abdominal muscles, I still couldn't hold my urine. More ominously, there were several times during my aerobics classes when I had the sensation that my towel was bunched up under my stomach as I lay on the floor, but when I looked at the towel, it was flat. Something, however, was there, something that was not a part of me and which seemed to occupy the space below my navel.

I called during the first week of August to make another appointment because I wanted you to check the persistent hardness stretching across my abdomen. Even when I protested that I thought I should see you immediately, I couldn't get an appointment until the last week in August. The hardness in my abdomen worried me, especially since my immediate plans to go to school meant giving up my job and health insurance. I knew that by the time late August arrived I would have assisted my employer in screening a replacement for me. My apartment would be in boxes because I had already given notice to my landlord. If the hardness in my abdomen should require surgery, I needed to know right away, not in three weeks. But how could I explain all of this to a hurried nurse of a doctor I had visited only twice? I was so frightened by the possibility of a tumor that I couldn't even talk about it to my best friends. I feared the worst, but again I waited.

And sure enough, it was the worst. After six months of viewing my symptoms as isolated and disconnected minor problems, suddenly you saw them as symptoms of only one thing: a tumor. For a change, I got fast action. On Friday I met with you, on the following Monday I had an ultrasound, and on Tuesday I had a CT scan, and on Wednesday I met with the surgeon. On Thursday and Friday, between pre-admission tests, I cancelled all plans for the future, and on Saturday, after five and a half hours in surgery, I woke up for a tiny second in post-op hearing my soul scream at the vision of my abdomen scooped out and bloodily exposed from one hip bone to the other.

The next time I woke up I was in my hospital room. Through the haze of anesthesia, I picked up the ringing telephone beside my bed and heard my surgeon tell me that with the benefit of chemotherapy and radiation I had—at best—a 40 percent chance of surviving this metastasized ovarian cancer. The chemotherapy would start in a matter of days, she said, just as soon as they removed the catheter. A football-sized tumor, the worst the assisting gynecological oncologist had ever seen, had been removed from my gut. Both of my ovaries, indistinguishable from the multi-chambered tumor, had been removed. For good measure my surgeon also removed my uterus, my fallopian tubes, my appendix, my omentum (a membrane passing between certain soft internal organs in the abdominal cavity), and the unique birthmark I favored which formerly rested inside my belly button. My bladder, the surgeon happened to remark, had been flattened to the thinness of a tortilla. Failing muscle tone, my ass.

With surprising fortitude, I accepted that I was going to die. I felt an odd sense of gratitude mixed with relief—gratitude that I had had my chance to live and relief that the challenge was over. It didn't matter anymore if I didn't pass the test. No one passes this one. Everyone dies.

Before the surgery, I had been grasping at goals just to have one to live for, but now my dreams of school and a new life seemed contrived. I spent much of the next two days looking at my life through a rear-view mirror. There was nothing ahead but a dead-end sign glaring me in the face. Then, with their tails between their legs, your colleagues came to tell me that the 40 percent survival prognosis given to me was wrong.

After closer examination of my tumor cells, the hospital pathologists couldn't agree on whether I even had full-blown cancer. The younger pathologists said no, the older ones said yes.

The messy, gelatin-like slides of my tumor were sent to specialists around the country. No one responded with any urgency, so the hospital tumor committee decided to give me no treatment. They would just observe my case. On the day I had scheduled my "New Lease on Life" party to celebrate this good news with my friends, I received a letter from one specialist saying that while no studies had been done on my form of cancer, certain aspects of my cells were quite foreboding. He concluded that I should try chemotherapy, even though chemotherapy probably wouldn't work. By this time I was beginning to have some doubts about the prognostic capabilities of Western medicine.

I had yet to complete the transition from accepting death to regaining hope for living. But as soon as I realized I would survive for at least the near future, I recognized what a mess I was in, and my mind turned to more practical things. The delay in my initial appointment with you to check the hardness in my abdomen—during which time I had resigned from my job—caused me to nearly lose my health insurance. That health insurance had already been worth $20,000 to me for the week in the hospital alone. In the two days between diagnosis and surgery, I had called my boss on his vacation and asked him for my job back. He had already offered my job to a person I had helped select, and she had already accepted, even though I hadn't yet turned the job over to her. But my boss assured me that although he couldn't give me my job back, he would work something out. He scraped together a temporary, lower-paying job for me.

I set about trying to repair my life. I had no idea what I wanted to look for in the way of a job because I had been so committed to a major career change before you finally discovered the tumor. My plans to become a student, living on the fringe economically with little security and sparse health coverage, were now out of the question. I became obsessed with health insurance. I was convinced I needed a job that offered sufficient wages to cover all the copayments I had accrued, that offered a health insurance policy with an immediate effective date and with no exclusions for pre-existing conditions, and that offered low stress so as not to aggravate my cancerous condition. I failed at every job interview, probably because I was convinced that the word "cancer" was carved in scarlet letters across my forehead.

I remained in the temporary job I had. Then, since nine months of ongoing tests had all yielded negative results, I began to think that perhaps I would stay in remission. Perhaps I could begin to take chances again, live again, dream again.

I worked very hard at my job to prove my new position should become permanent so that I could maintain my health insurance. Then I started feeling sick again. First it was "just a cold," but your associate—in your absence—warned me to call back in a week if it hadn't cleared up. It did not clear up. Instead I started getting infections in all the places that had been affected by my metastasized cancer: the bladder, the intestines, the vagina and the anus. It hurt to urinate, my swollen vagina itched intensely, there were sores around my anus, and my intestines were distended and hard. I began vomiting, and my bowel movements were loose and irregular. I remembered the tiny bits of cancer, the "grains of sand," which had been left on my intestines after the surgery. I kept thinking about how, for a while after the surgery, there had been "communication" between my abdominal cavity and my vagina; my cervix had not completely closed after the surgery, and there was some possibility that the cancer cells which remained in my abdominal cavity could have been carried through the cervix into the vagina where they might take up housekeeping.

I had learned my lesson. This time I listened to my body. I tried to identify what was wrong with my whole system instead of focusing on isolated symptoms. I thought it probable that my cancer was invading the remaining abdominal organs, thus causing all these infections. And of course, I was panic-stricken.

I called you when the infections first began, but I wasn't even allowed to talk to you because, after all, "it was only a cold." When I had become sufficiently scared to call your office, I wanted to see you and no one else. I thought you would know best the dangers of treating each of these symptoms as an isolated incident, since we had made that mistake before. You knew my body now, and you knew that when I say there is something wrong, I am not being just a hypochondriac.

So when your nurse said I had to go to the emergency room to see you, I went. Dressed in a hospital gown with a hospital name tag fastened to my wrist, I sat on a gurney and waited for you for two hours, becoming more and more fearful. Finally I was told you had called and directed that I be seen by another doctor. I called your office to verify this message, and the answering service responded that your office was closed for lunch. Upon my insistence, the answering service said they'd have you call me back. The answering service apologetically called me back themselves to say that I simply must see another doctor, and that was that.

The last thing I wanted was to have some strange male doctor who was totally unfamiliar with my case insert and open a speculum in my burning vagina until I screamed in pain, ask me about my last menstrual period, and then tell me that I looked healthy to him and that a little daily dab of estrogen cream should solve all my problems. Experience had made me distrustful, and rather than risk suffering such an indignity, I left the emergency room, disgusted with the medical system.

I went into the hospital cafeteria, and there I ran into you. I was angry, and I let you know it. I can understand your defensiveness; I would have been defensive, too, if I were you. But when you told me that I should be grateful that I had received as much care as I had, and that in comparison to your AIDS patients I was not that badly off, I saw once again that I could expect a quick response from you only if you feared I might die then and there, right at your feet. I knew at that moment that for the sake of my life my relationship with you had to be severed.

Still, I honestly don't believe that you are responsible for the myriad health care problems I've had. All the obstacles I have encountered can be seen, when it comes down to the bottom line, as symptoms of a health care system that is faltering on the brink of disaster. The day I saw you in the cafeteria you looked exhausted, overworked, and desperate. When any physician has more patients than there are days in the year, he or she can't possibly give the kind of care of which I know you are capable.

This situation is not fair to you, and it's not fair to me nor to anyone else—workers or clients—in the health care system. Health care quality and accessibility in our country varies dramatically in different hospitals and with different insurance plans. The enormous paperwork and record-keeping and bill-sending bureaucracy to which we all are slaves takes up the bulk of health care time and energy; it is no wonder that physicians can't keep up with the latest developments or the implications of the latest techniques. A friend of mine who went to a public hospital had to wait a whole month for her ultrasound results before she could have surgery for ovarian cancer. Her doctor told her after her surgery that she could still have children, and in the same breath he told her that she would need radiation treatments. The radiation plunged her into instant menopause. I suppose it's possible that he really didn't know.

I was more fortunate than my friend; I was operated on within four days of my diagnosis, and my post-surgical treatment was thoroughly debated. But had I been enrolled in an HMO at that time, my tumor slides might never have been sent to the national experts who would not have been "member physicians." If those experts had not recommended against further treatment, I might have needlessly undergone the miseries of radiation and chemotherapy.

But even though I felt my choices would be severely limited by an HMO, I finally decided that I had to join one. After my surgery I was forced to limit my job search to big employers because small businesses can usually afford only less complete health coverage, and small business employees are also often excluded from federal regulations which protect employees from health insurance rate hikes from conversion to an individual plan for eighteen months after they leave the company. My insurance, which costs my employer $150 per month at the group rate, would have cost me $500 per month as an individual. Since my job after my surgery was only a temporary one, I felt I had to switch to an HMO so that I could afford the individual premium when I am laid off.

Now that I am in an HMO, I don't have to face the probability of $500-per-month premiums, but I am enmeshed in the bewildering tangle of an entrenched bureaucracy. I must have a CT scan every six months for the next three years, but before I can make an appointment for a scan, a request in writing has to be made by my primary care physician to the HMO. Then I must wait for a letter of approval from the HMO administrators. Every three months I must visit the gynecologist for my pelvic exam, and then I must get an appointment with my oncologist, who is the only one capable of interpreting the results of the CT scan and blood tests. Lastly, I have to see the primary care physician, who must request authorization for all of it. Each physician bills at $80 for a five-minute visit. It's difficult to decide whom I should call for my scan and test results; the primary care physician is only able to interpret the results in general and not very useful terms, but the hospital can't send the results to anyone other than the primary care physician who orders the tests in the first place.

My oncologist discourages me from visiting my gynecological

oncologist, who is not a "member" physician of the HMO to which I belong. Yet my gynecologist will not make a move without consulting that very same gynecological oncologist whom she had invited to be the assisting physician in my surgery; he is the recognized expert. This gynecological oncologist has his own office and is in so much demand that it's not in his interests to belong to an HMO. My HMO does not have a gynecological oncologist. The HMO apparently prefers to pay three member-physicians to see me quarterly instead of paying just one—the gynecological oncologist.

The physicians in the HMOs are frustrated. They are too over-worked to keep up on medical developments, and that forces me to spend hours poring over medical journals with a dictionary so that I can get the answers I need in order to make rational decisions. My HMO oncologist spends part of my half-hour appointments telling me about how hard he works and that he still can't afford to redo his kitchen. Unable to afford the more prestigious private offices, he shares an office in a busy medical building adjacent to the hospital. He claims that his first forty hours each week go just to cover his overhead, and that my HMO reimburses him at rates lower than their "market value" after they charged him $2,000 to join the HMO.

I don't know how much commiseration I feel for the financial problems of my oncologist, but for all of the above reasons I do have some sympathy for you as another doctor in this insane system. I regret that I'm forced to search elsewhere for the kind of service I must have in order to fight for my life, because I feel you could have provided it had you had the time. I don't have much faith that I will find an improvement anywhere until some drastic changes are made in our nation's health care system. I may live to see those changes, or I may not. In the meantime, I will live whatever is left of my life with the fear that one of those grains of sand will grow to the size of a football again, just waiting for a drop in my defenses to get itself going.

Nuclear Medicine Clinic

SUSAN EISENBERG

All the comfortable chairs, the bouquets
the coffee tables with magazines are
upstairs in the maternity wing where
curtained windows open out to the sky.

Here, in the basement bunker, where those who
touch us wear special rings and badges,
where medication is stored behind lead shields
there are no windows or magazines

only a palpable fear
of flowers.

No cheerful team of nurses welcomes
us, only a receptionist who asks after our
insurance, then directs us to hard plastic seats
where we wait to be called by name.

With stolen glances, we inspect each other
then compute our place in the line-ups of
age and luck. No one asks friendly questions
or even smiles.   We keep politely

silent, hoping for news that is
not bad.

When the Cure Becomes the Cause

NITA RABINOVITCH

An iatrogenic disorder is an illness arising from treatment prescribed by a physician. According to *Churchill's Medical Dictionary*, the term "iatrogenic" means "pertaining to or describing a complication, injury, unfavorable result or other problem which can be directly attributed to medical care." Like most people, I was unaware of this medical phenomenon. Today I am all too aware. I have an iatrogenic cancer.

People go to doctors when they are sick because they expect the doctors to make them well. But for all of its pretensions toward infallibility, the practice of medicine in many ways is still primitive and at times inept. Oncology is a good example. Now that cancer has become such a widespread and common disease, millions of people go to doctors to be treated for cancer, and many of those people will tell you that the treatment for cancer seemed a great deal worse than the disease. Still, many of those people will be helped by the treatment, even though the treatment may make them feel much sicker than the disease did. More and more evidence is coming to light, however, that the current treatments for cancer are not only unpleasant, they are often downright dangerous in and of themselves and too often even cause a cancer when they were administered to treat a cancer.

My personal introduction to cancer happened in 1975, when an innocent-appearing cyst in my left breast took on some not-so-benign characteristics. My surgeon, who had been following the cyst with manual examination and mammograms, said, "It's almost certain to be nothing; we'll do a biopsy next week, and in the unlikely event that the frozen section shows it to be malignant, we'll do a mastectomy while you're still under anesthesia."

My reaction to that plan was immediate. "No," I said. "We'll not do a mastectomy; we'll just do a biopsy, and if it should be malignant, I'll get information about all possible treatments and then decide."

As I think back, I am surprised now by my response. I was not the assertive type, and consumer advocacy in medicine had not yet become customary or even acceptable. The single procedure of following a biopsy with a mastectomy was routine in those days.

My surgeon explained the disadvantages to my plan. First, he said, it would require anesthesia twice instead of once. Secondly, disturbance of the tissue during the biopsy could dislodge some cancerous cells which might then travel within my body, set up housekeeping in a new place, and become the start of a metastatic lesion. I stuck to my guns, in part because I could not face the double threat of cancer and mastectomy, and I decided to put off worrying about it until I knew for sure with what we were dealing.

The following week I entered the hospital in the late afternoon. When I was presented with the surgery permission form to sign, I read it thoroughly, and I was troubled by some of the loose language (for example, "I authorize my physician to perform any other procedure that in his judgment is advisable for my well-being"). I added to "biopsy—left breast" my own handwritten words, "biopsy only! no mastectomy!" The nurse who watched me add my own words to the consent form was amazed. She explained to me that such changes on the form had never been made before, and she thought I should rethink my position.

But I was optimistic. I was sure that I housed no malignancy. Nevertheless, I was crystal clear that if my lump should turn out to be cancerous, I wanted the time and opportunity to weigh all the alternatives and prepare myself psychologically should I opt for a mastectomy. I learned much later that my independent behavior caused quite a ripple of alarm in the hospital staff.

I don't remember much of that morning when I underwent the biopsy. My first distinct memory is of being roused while I was in the recovery room by my surgeon. "Nita," he was saying, "it was malignant." Even in my drugged state, the regret in his voice came through to me.

Once I gained full consciousness, I became intent on exploring the alternatives I had not wanted to think about before the biopsy. The surgeon advised a mastectomy, but I had read in my favorite medical journal, *Time* magazine, about the new procedure of lumpectomy followed by radiation. The term lumpectomy can mean either a wide excision in which the tumor and a margin of normal tissue surrounding it are removed, leaving both the skin and underlying muscle intact, or the simpler tumor excision in which only the tumor is removed. I knew lumpectomies were being performed in the eastern part of the United States and that lumpectomy was a common procedure for early breast cancer in Europe. Since the whole tumor had been excised during my biopsy, the procedure performed on me had been similar to a lumpectomy. The five-year survival rate for mastectomy and lumpectomy was the same; the ten-year survival rate was 15 percent better with mastectomy. It seemed to me that with the enormous drive and financial support being given to cancer research and treatment, it was likely that a cure might be just around the corner. Though my surgeon would never have initiated a discussion about radiation with me, the combination of survival statistics, my expectation of real breakthroughs in cancer treatment, and my desire to avoid the mutilation and pain of surgery all led me to decide that I should see an expert in radiation therapy.

I made an appointment with a radiation therapist for the next week. The radiation therapist confirmed the statistics regarding survival but also told me that the target population who received radiation instead of mastectomy were usually those whom surgeons considered incurable by surgery because their tumors were too advanced. These patients were therefore not a true control group, but were instead a skewed sample. If that were true, I reasoned, then radiation therapy—for me, with a small tumor—should give me an even better chance at ten-year survival. I asked about possible side effects. I was told that radiation would make further lactation in the irradiated breast impossible. At the age of forty-six, with three children, ages fourteen, seventeen, and twenty-two, I found the inability to breast-feed an acceptable loss.

I remember that I felt some embarrassment, but also some amusement, when the doctor drew what appeared to be a crazy road map in green on my chest—markers to guide the technician in directing the cobalt machine and placing the lead shields. I even had permanent dye spots tattooed on me (I never thought I was the tattoo type). For nine weeks I received radiation treatments daily except for weekends. Everyone at the clinic was helpful, kind, and eager to make my treatments as convenient as possible. I was scheduled to be radiated at noon, and I drove from my work to the Health Sciences Center on my lunch hour, got "zapped," and drove back to my office eating a sandwich and an apple which I had packed that morning. Continuing with my normal schedule was my way of coping; I didn't miss a beat. All in all, I missed only one day of work. In retrospect, I'm not sure that was the best way to handle it.

When I reached the five-year mark with no metastasis, I thought I was home free. I was cured of cancer, and I had emerged intact, with no mutilation. I had beaten the odds.

Then in February of 1986—more than ten years after I had been diagnosed with cancer—I began feeling pain in my left shoulder and some numbness in my left hand. The pain got worse and worse. X-rays were taken, but they showed nothing. Wearing a sling and consuming great quantities of aspirin, I went back and forth from surgeon to radiologist to neurosurgeon to find some explanation for the pain and numbness. Three difficult and frightening weeks after my first X-ray, another X-ray was taken. This one showed a fracture in my clavicle. We assumed that the fracture was caused by radiation damage resulting in a general weakening of the bone irradiated during the breast cancer treatments.

But my clavicle never knit. Six months after the fracture was discovered, the orthopedist, upon examining successive X-rays and noting that bone cells were not building up but instead seemed to be disappearing, became suspicious that there might be a malignancy and recommended a biopsy. The doctors were reluctant to do a biopsy, however, because irradiated tissue heals so poorly, and if the biopsy area should become infected the poorly vascularized tissue would not supply enough white cells to fight the infection.

But by November, when there still had been no improvement, everyone was nervous enough to risk a needle biopsy. The results were inconclusive. In December we tried again, and again the results were inconclusive. Finally, in February—a full year after the fracture—an open biopsy was performed. This time they took enough tissue to get results, and at last there was a diagnosis. I had a radiation-induced sarcoma (a malignant fibrous histiocytoma), unrelated to the breast cancer itself but caused by the radiation treatments. I began to acquire a familiarity with medical terms I really never wished to learn about.

The treatment for my iatrogenic cancer was to remove the left clavicle in which the tumor was embedded. However, since that entire area had received such massive radiation twelve years earlier, we knew that an incision of that sort would never heal. So a plan was devised to use muscle tissue from my back to graft onto my upper chest wall to cover the opening made in removing my clavicle. This "major, major" surgery (as my "major, major" surgeon put it) was performed by two teams of experts. The first team was headed by an orthopedic oncologist who separated me from my malignant bone. The second team was headed by a plastic surgeon who used my latissimus dorsi muscle and an enormous skin graft from my thigh to cover the gaping hole in my upper chest.

I don't remember much of that surgery. I was heavily drugged, and besides reducing my pain, the medication also obliterated my memory. My family, who spent many hours with me, were not quite so lucky; they weren't medicated and could be fully aware of what was going on. For one of my daughters the visits to my bedside must have been particularly grim; her husband, who had died one month earlier from a brain tumor, had received treatment in the same hospital.

I didn't have much energy, but I needed some focus outside of myself. I went back to work a month after the surgery. I wore a special sling which immobilized my shoulder and arm so that the rearrangement of my body accomplished in the surgery would have a chance to become permanent.

Physical therapy helped. One can function quite well without a clavicle, though there is loss of strength. I was not prepared, however, for the progressive numbness in my left hand which I had first felt at the time of the original fracture. What had been only a minor problem then has now become a major disability. Apparently the radiation not only had caused the cancer in my clavicle, it had also damaged nerves in my brachial plexus, the network of nerves which go to the arm and hand. My left hand now functions like a weak paw. It has lost all its strength and dexterity and can no longer grasp anything. The old expression, "losing one's grip," has dramatic meaning to me now. Any two-handed operations, like tying shoes or cutting up food with a knife and fork, are extremely difficult.

When I was first diagnosed with breast cancer and chose radiation as treatment, I kept my cancer a secret. My family knew, of course, and I told a few close friends and my supervisor at work. I was afraid I would be treated differently, that people might avoid me because they would fear contagion or because I aroused too much anxiety in them. Nor did I want overly solicitous sympathy. Also I feared that the fact of my cancer might hurt future employment; I didn't want any prospective employer to be swayed by a concern about my dependability or insurance cost.

But when the cancer in my shoulder—a side effect of the treatment for the first cancer—appeared, I did not keep it a secret this time. The outpouring of love and attention from friends and colleagues has been a major healing experience, and it has demonstrated for me that secrecy would have been a major mistake, for it would have denied me some very precious support and help.

That love and support from family and friends continues to be crucial. Unfortunately, the tumor, it turned out, was not confined to my clavicle, and in less than three months after the surgery I had a recurrence of the tumor in my neck. This tumor was removed with a very minor excision, but a month later I had a recurrence of the recurrence. Again we tried an excision, but when the tumor reappeared we knew surgery was not the answer. At this point, I took a six-month leave of absence from my work and ultimately had to resign. In the two and a half years since these surgeries, I have tried chemotherapy, using at various times two or three of five different major drugs. It is a very stubborn tumor in a very stubborn host. My latest battle plan has been the interstitial implantation of radioisotopes which we hope will retard the growth of the tumor. It might even be a cure. During all this time I have used meditation, humor, and as many of the psychological techniques as I can to strengthen my ability to fight the disease and improve my life.

I am keenly aware of the iatrogenic nature of my present illness. Every time I try a new experimental treatment, or even a "tried and true" one, I am aware that I may be letting myself in for side effects that may be worse than the illness itself. My most difficult occupation these days is the risk/benefit analysis in which I must make judgments and decisions without adequate information; there just isn't enough known. Though the treatments I choose to have may make me a statistic, I cannot know until I try them if I shall fall into that class for which the treatment will be a success or a disaster.

For instance, I considered and decided to try Cisplatin (a chemotherapeutic agent), even though it carried the risk of several side effects. I did suffer the effect of some mild hearing loss and some nerve damage in my feet, which makes me a bit unsteady and gives me the feeling that my shoes are full of sand. I counter this disability with medication which relieves some of the tingling in my feet and left hand but which has its own side effect—a dry mouth. I combat the dry mouth by sucking candy, but I fear that this sugary solution will be detrimental to my teeth. My teeth are more important to me than most other people's are to them; I need my teeth not just for chewing, but I need them also to dress myself. There are often times when I feel quite trapped in my own Catch-22.

There has been one other noteworthy side effect of my cancer. That is the bills. Bills, insurance claims and EOBs (explanation of benefits) constitute a sizable part of my mail. Even if all of the bills were accurate, they are complex enough to occupy a full-time accountant who is healthy. However, the bills are frequently inaccurate. Insurance companies make mistakes, and secondary carriers are often confused. Communications get lost as they go from one desk to another. It takes tremendous work to ensure that health care providers are paid their proper fees by one's primary and secondary insurers so that the patient pays appropriate deductibles and co-insurance. This is not a job for a sick person.

I recognize that my decision to choose radiation therapy rather than mastectomy was a mistake, but it was *I* who made that decision. Though I have deeply regretted my decision, I have never beat my chest with guilt (it's too tender, anyway). At the time, the choice I made definitely seemed the right thing to do. The medical profession is only now beginning to recognize the potential dangers from all forms of ionizing radiation, and the medical literature is just beginning to reflect the recent realization that therapeutic radiation can do as much harm as good.

"First do no harm" is a basic tenet of the Hippocratic oath, an ancient pledge traditionally taken by graduating physicians when they complete medical school. This basic tenet recognizes that treatment has the potential to do injury and that the esteem in which the physician is held gives her or him special power over the patient. In the complexity of modern medicine, both physicians and patients must frequently make critical decisions balancing potential cure against possible harm. The more serious the disease, the greater the willingness to undergo unpleasant, even dangerous, treatment. When the harm of a particular treatment is delayed in time or is not the usual outcome, physicians may find out too late that they have unwittingly done a patient far more harm than good. And though the doctor may have to live with the responsibility, it is the patient who must live with, or die from, "the cure."

Letter to My Mother

APRIL LINDNER

On doctor's orders you took to the guest bed
and in your satin housecoat, your pink hair ribbon,
waited out the dangerous pregnancy, your first,
thumbing through movie magazines
for baby names.   Each day the sun
passed from the east
to the west window and each night the moon
anchored itself above your bed.

Did you sleep?   Or were the weeks
broken only by breakfast, lunch, supper
taken like high mass, the tumbler
of buttermilk: *let my child be well,*
dish of spinach: *let my child be strong,*
and one white pill every night
set on your tongue like communion:
let my child be born.   When the doctor

gave you the good news—finally pregnant—
he handed you the prescription slip
and you squinted to make out
his hieroglyphic wisdom.   I was born
into his palms, screamed my surprise
in the bright room, and he pronounced me
perfectly symmetrical, but why do I tell
this story back to you who told it first to me?

not to blame you, not even to blame
that doctor, ten years dead,
who believed each pill was a small
white miracle, who believed himself
a good man, handing out babies like gifts
wrapped in pastel blankets.   No, I can't
hate you or him or even hate
my own doctor who, eyes averted, says
I'm not symmetrical at all, says my insides

are ingrown, I'm barely fit to carry
babies of my own.   I never was perfect,
not even in your sweet womb, mother,
the rich red guest room that locked out
raw oxygen, harsh light, traffic noises
but not the poison that leaked
through the cord we shared.   Those pills
filtered in, invaded the pulsing nubs.

my veins, seeped into my blood,
I bloomed awry, each new cell stuck

to the others by thick white glue.
So we learn the truth: love is imperfect,
no protection, and the houses we build
to keep each other safe are delicate
as the nests of wasps, dissolve
like paper in the rain.

Editor's note: The drug referred to in this poem is DES (diethylstilbestrol), a synthetic estrogen approved by the Food and Drug Administration in 1942 and prescribed for millions of pregnant women between 1941 and 1971 who had a history of miscarriage, high blood pressure, diabetes, or slight bleeding. Use of the drug was stopped when it was discovered that daughters of women who took DES were more likely to develop cancers of the vagina and cervix. See *The New Our Bodies, Ourselves*, by the Boston Women's Health Book Collective, Simon & Schuster, New York, 1984, for more information.

IV. Living in Our Bodies: Cancer, Self-Image and Sexuality

Letter to Lisa in California

APRIL LINDNER

In the bare middle of the night flip
the bathroom switch and catch your face
framed by the mirror, sharp

chin, dark crackle of hair, eyes
luminous and green, soon eclipsed
by the moon of my face. I was new

at school, the one you wanted
to like, and people confused us,
called me Lisa sometimes,

called you April. Is that why
he wanted us both, first you
then me? You blamed me

as I do, riding off
in his white Pontiac, bare feet
propped on the dashboard, September

sun in my eyes, him taking corners
too fast. Who knew that sleek trophy,
that penis we spat sparks over, shot death

with each sweet clot of cream? Condyloma!
Lovely name, like Cinderella or
Rumpelstiltskin. Condyloma,

name the doctors taught me
for invisible warts that crawl
up the long tunnel in search of someplace

moist and dark. Now they bloom and bloom,
purple buds, and the ache that spread
low and hot is from doctors

snipping spoiled flesh like bruises
from a peach, doctors prodding
and telling each other—

like I wasn't there, the inquisitor's
lamp burning my legs—that they want
my uterus, want to save me

from my uterus. Lisa,
I imagine you in California
awake beside your sleeping husband,

pregnant and stroking your muskmelon belly,
Lisa, I stand naked in the courtroom
before the jury, twelve of you, I point

to my sutures, the black thread
like barbed wire, I spread my palms
to show I carry no weapons

and I say, too late,
it is each other we should love.

Making It

JACKIE MANTHORNE

"Would you like to dance?"

I turn and look at you. Our eyes connect immediately, and I think how unusual it is to see somebody else my age here. But that and your lovely, lively eyes and your smiling face aren't enough to penetrate my defenses.

"Not really."

"Why not?" you ask, your eyes still twinkling with infinite possibilities.

Why do you want to know? Why aren't you like the rest of those women who melt away into the smoky shadows when they feel me slam the door in their faces? Cruising dykes don't have much confidence; on the other hand, it seems that you might have too much. I decide that I don't like you.

"I'm not ready," I blurt. Shit! I meant to say something else, something that would fit my haughty look of dismissal, something that even you would recognize as rejection, and as final.

"You mean you're still getting over a relationship?"

Ah, the analytic older bar dyke. But can't you tell that I'm getting impatient? Don't you know that I don't owe you anything, especially answers? "Something like that." My response is wry: I'm thinking of my missing breast. Missing in action, as they say. Invaded by one of the cancers of our time. We had a relationship, me and my left tit, for fifty-five years. A real, solid, substantial one—both the relationship and the tit, actually. And I miss it.

"Well, let's sit this one out and have a drink together," you suggest, interrupting my slightly maudlin musings on the state of my chest.

I find that I don't mind sitting with you. After all, I can be alone even if we're sharing a table. Your physical presence is only a slight annoyance, mainly because I've noticed how attractive you are, and some of those old urges I thought were dead and buried seem to be very much alive. Old habits die hard.

If you could read my thoughts, you would think that I've given up. I'm sure that would remove the purposeful gleam from your eyes and send you off to more fertile corners of the bar. But if I wanted to, I would tell you that I haven't given up, I haven't succumbed to that limbo state of being a cancer victim. Temptation surrounded me from the first day. My doctor baited me by being kind; hospital workers set traps with their every sympathetic word and gesture; the loss of my hair and the nausea from being cooked with radiation and spiced with toxic chemicals exhorted me to become one of "them"—the sick, the maimed, the doomed. But I've been one of "them" all my life, first as a woman, then as a lesbian, and I've had lots of practice at passing, until finally I made a conscious choice not to pass. And since then I've become quite adept at fighting back when I can and ignoring it when I can't.

But I wasn't able to ignore my missing breast, and neither was my lover of ten years. She left less than a year later for rather vague reasons which I was tempted to believe because the truth was harder to take. It wasn't that she wanted a "whole" woman; I don't think she really minded that I only had one breast, even though she had always joked that she was a "boob lady." No, it was more than that. I think she just couldn't stand the thought that cancer cells might still be frolicking around inside my body, deciding in what nourishing spot to set up housekeeping and have a second go at killing me. She couldn't stand the waiting, the suspense, the agony of not knowing. So she ran right to the other side of the continent, and all I have left of her is a box of photos of happier, more naive times. And once in a while she sends me a postcard, but it never says, "Wish you were here."

That was over a year ago, and those scars have healed. I'm not even bitter about it any more. Or so I think. But why should I trust you? I see health streaming from your eyes, radiating from your pores, in the tilt of your head, in your foot-stomping reaction to the beat of the music. You are alive and healthy and you know it; you've never had a reason to doubt it. What's more, you think that you have the right to be alive and healthy, and that makes me fear you.

"Want to talk about it?" you ask.

"Not really," I reply evenly.

"Want to talk about something else, then?"

I laugh; you are persistent, and I rather like that in a woman. So I decide to make it easy on you, and start talking about nothing much: the weather, current trends in music, movies I've seen, others I'd like to see. You quickly realize that I'm being very cautious, and you don't try to take our conversation deeper. I feel a sense of relief that you're satisfied with chit-chat, at least for the moment, and I start to relax. After all, it's Friday night at the bar, I'm sitting here with an attractive woman, and if my memory serves me right, that's a very appropriate, normal thing for me to be doing.

So after a while I let you talk me into dancing, and it feels good to be moving with the music, facing you, watching you watch me. And when you put your arms around me for a slow dance, I'm not too nervous to appreciate the warmth or the strength or the comfort or the sexiness of your body. It's been a long time, too long. But how does a one-breasted woman cruise? How does she overcome the loss of an important part of her body and the threat of cancer and the reaction of a prospective lover? How does she find other lesbians her own age when every year the women in the bars seem younger?

I listen to you whisper in my ear, inviting me home. Poor you, I think as I accept, you're getting more than you bargained for. Or less, depending on how you think about it. Can I trust you not to hurt me? Perhaps I'll have to start learning how not to be hurt by what others can't accept. I feel very attracted to you and I want to act on that feeling; I want to remember that I'm alive and sexy and sexual.

The drive to your house in the suburbs is long but not uncomfortable. You tell me about your middle management job in a large company, you entertain me with stories about how you bought your house and about all the things which have gone wrong since day one, you scatter bits and pieces of information about your former relationships here and there to keep me interested. I tell you nothing, and you respect my silence. Or perhaps you like shy, quiet women.

I am sitting on your bed as you pour wine into two glasses which you then place on the bedside table. I'm not ready, not in the least, but I'm miles away from the safety of my own home.

"Whatever possessed you to buy a house out here?" I ask, as you hand me a glass and sit beside me.

You laugh. "A big back yard, cleaner air, less noise. I find I can pretend that I actually live in the country."

Your arms go around me and you nuzzle my neck, sending shivers through my body.

"Do you live in the city?" you ask, your hands exploring.

I nod, not trusting my voice. I want to turn and bury my face in your flesh, but I can't. I want to run from your bed and from your house and most of all from your enticing lips and arms and body, but I can't. I am concentrating on not spilling my wine, but that's not the main reason why I can't move, and finally I feel my eyes closing and the wine glass being taken from my hand, and then you are easing me back on the bed and kissing me gently, your hands moving over me, removing my clothing, and I panic as my bra falls away and with it my prosthesis.

"Ah," you breathe, and for a moment you stare down at me silently. I open my eyes, afraid but needing to look at you. Your face is flushed with desire, and as I watch you reach out and lightly slide your fingers over my breast, then repeat the gesture over my scar. Only then do you look at me and smile.

"I . . ."

You place a finger over my lips. "Later." Your mouth replaces your finger and your kiss is soft, but I feel the heat, the need in the trembling of your body, and I know I want you very, very much. I groan and pull you to me hard, my mouth opening. I want it all, I want you all, and I don't want to wait any more.

Dracula Meets a Chemo-Poet

HELENE DAVIS

Dracula comes through my window, hungry as usual. Fine, I say, hungry too, hungry for the kiss, the bite, everlasting life. He shows up in his rented suit and fine white shirt. He is wearing his company manners. "Would you be so kind," he says. "Yes." And I picture his wings protecting me in the dark skies. Dracula drinks my blood and vomits six hours later. In three weeks he loses all his hair.

Construction

ANNA SHALER

The first man I slept with after the breakup with Michael couldn't think of anything he wanted me to cook him for dinner except steak. I don't eat meat, only fish and chicken sometimes. I told him I could make a wonderful fish dinner and asked him what he'd like, or what he'd order in a lovely restaurant, and he said, "Fish sticks. I eat fish sticks."

I am not a snob, especially when it comes to men, even though I made this rule that I'd never again go out with any man who didn't know who Sir Ralph Richardson was. I got past that rule pretty quickly with Brendan. That's his name—Brendan, the most gorgeous name for a man I've ever heard. He told me some of the guys he worked with called him Brenda, and, boy, his cheeks turned pink when he laughed at himself. I said, "Didn't you ever hear of Brendan Behan, the great drunken Irish poet?"

He said, "No."

So what. He was looking down at me like a great big beacon of Gaelic sunlight, a pink-skinned blue-eyed open-faced Irish Catholic-boy construction worker who'd been dying to meet me for months and months while all I'd done was parade my brokenhearted self as best I could past his site several times a day. My plan had been to attract him by walking out my door any time between the hours of 7 a.m. and 3 p.m., pass by looking good, and catch the smile that came from him, hotter every day, just like the weather. It was safe to smile back at him; there were no catcalls, no sucking noises or remarks of any kind from his co-workers, and so we reached the next level of our affair by adding a wave of the hands. The fear that I would never be looked at again was totally assuaged.

The first time I said, "Hi," he turned bright red and stumbled backward. Later, I put him to a test to see if he really liked me, and so I walked by as though I'd forgotten he existed.

"Hey, Hi! Hey!" he shouted, jumping up and down on the

muddy platform like a cheerleader in his baseball cap and heavy boots. I turned my head.

"Oh, hi," I said. What a bitch. And I could do that all day long if I felt like it—strut and tease, parade myself back and forth proving anything I wanted to prove. Wounded, I welcomed a flirtation with a foreigner, nothing more.

The day he waved his gloved hand at me from the seventh story—an open square, as yet consisting only of steel girders and cement—I thought my heart would stop. He must have meant to do that to me, his chest smooth and bare, his blue-jeaned legs planted in the widest triangle his body would accommodate. He looked so strong and so very, very sweet up there.

The next day he crossed the street to come and speak to me.

"What are you doin'?" he asked.

"Nothing. Why?"

"Well, I'm Brendan."

"Hi, Brendan. My name's Madeleine. Maddy."

"Madeleine. It's nice to meet you."

I had to lean against the mailbox I had just put my week's work into. I saw his face flush pink to lavender to pink again, his laugh held tight so he wouldn't get the giggles. I was weak. I hadn't planned to get this intimate, although I wished like hell that Michael would walk out of his building and see me talking to this guy. Right after we broke up I had to watch him walk up and down the street with some pinheaded girl he was spending time with. Living across the street from your ex-boyfriend is hell, except when the opportunity arises to get even.

"Where are you goin'?" Brendan said.

"Nowhere. I came out to use the mailbox."

"This is the express box. What's your hurry?"

I told him that it was a script which had to get to California yesterday.

He laughed. "Like this building. We're two months behind schedule. But that's nothin' new. So, I saw you talkin' to the crane operator the other day. What was wrong, too noisy?"

"No," I said. "This noise isn't so bad. The noise when you were drilling rock for the foundation drove me crazy, but I don't mind the noise of the crane so much. I'm used to it. The problem is the exhaust from the diesel fuel. It comes in my window and makes my eyes burn, and, well, it's poison. I mean, we're not supposed to breathe that stuff. It's awful."

"Yeah, the noise. Well, his job will be finished soon."

"No, it's not the noise; it's the diesel exhaust. You see his stack there? It points right at my window. And it comes from the trucks, too, the ones that haul the wood and steel and stuff. The fumes are terrible . . ."

"Yeah, it's noisy," he said, grinning, his blue eyes two shutters taking pictures of my face. I could have been speaking Russian.

"So," he said. "You work?"

"Sure do. Right up there, right across from you."

"You work at home. So what do you do?"

"I write for TV. Daytime TV, in California. I mean, the show comes from California, so I mail it in."

"A writer." He nodded his approval. "I see you going in and out all day . . ."

"Yeah, I'm either going to the post office, the Xerox place, running errands, or walking around to clear my mind."

"That's good."

"How's your job?"

"Oh, it's good. I'm a shop steward. I clock the guys in and out and do whatever needs doing. It's a good job, a lot of money, not bad. I get to work in different places, get to meet interesting people. Nice people." He paused. I was the "nice people" he was talking about. My heart was knocking at the inside of my chest, climbing up a ladder to a pulse point in my neck. I was adorable, there was no doubt about it, and where the hell was Michael?

"This is a great neighborhood," Brendan said, shifting his weight from one foot to the other. "So. Do you go out? I mean, in the neighborhood?"

I looked down, then up at him, not knowing which of the two questions to answer. Or even whether it was two questions or one.

"Sometimes . . . sure."

"Well, I'll see you, then. In the neighborhood."

"See you."

I went home. I didn't even know whether I went out or not. I had been with Michael for seven years. I was alone now. Of course I went out in the neighborhood. Was Brendan asking me out, or what? I wanted to know. Since the breakup with Michael I was an egomaniac with no self-esteem.

And what about your body, Maddy? He doesn't know you're damaged. Oh, for chrissakes, he's just told you his name, and already you've got him feeling for your tits. You don't have to worry what it would be like with someone new; you're not up to that yet.

Brendan was buying beer and sandwiches for the guys when I stepped into the deli. I saw him through the window and walked in with a boldness born of my morning's depression at the thought of Michael across the street in his little apartment with some new girlfriend's contact lens solution in his medicine chest. Earlier I'd stood in line at the bank for twenty-five minutes with rock and roll turned up so loud on my earphones that others on the line recoiled from the audio overflow.

"What're you doin' here?" Brendan said when he saw me.

"I came in to see you." No pink and lavender this time. His face turned red as a beet with the greens still on.

"Brendan," I said.

He laughed, tipping his cap and throwing his head back, and looked over at the beer and then at me. "That's me. How's your writing?"

"Fine."

"Taking a break, huh?"

I nodded.

"Walk me to the Chinese place, then."

We were getting somewhere. It was almost like a date, walking down the street side by side with a common destination. Brendan had this cute way of shifting all of his weight from one foot to the other as he walked. I was breathless and found a way almost immediately to use the word "ex-boyfriend." We were talking about car radios as we passed by Brendan's brand new black and red four-by-four parked nearby.

"I don't have a radio in my car any more," I said. "It was stolen on the last day my ex-boyfriend used it. Isn't it funny how everything goes bad at once?"

"No radio? We'll have to get you a new one. I know some people; I'll see what I can do."

It sounded good to me.

I watched him take money out of his wallet, dig for change in the tight pocket of his jeans and pay for the egg rolls and fried rice. We turned away from the Chinese man behind the counter, facing each other in the tiny takeout store.

"So," he said. "Do you go out . . . in the neighborhood?"

"Sure."

"So if I called you on a Friday night, would you meet me for a drink?"

"I don't know. I might." I laughed. I also wrote my number down on the green Chinese receipt.

"Okay, so I'll see you in the neighborhood."

"Okay."

It was Wednesday, two days away from my first date since the one with Michael that had lasted seven years. I counted on my fingers the months since I had last been loved. It was ten. I counted ten.

On Friday morning Brendan called. His voice sounded confident, playful. Would I meet him?

"Yes."

I counted on my fingers the years since my body had been whole. Four. Four years ago an X-ray picture found cancer in my breast, the left one.

My breasts were sweet and tiny, the kind you would never think anything would happen to. They were perfect for my body, and I loved them even though the nipples were too pointy. When I got the news I hung up the phone, cried out and called Michael. He was there, across the street, not knowing.

"Michael," I said in a teeny little voice. "It's cancer, I have a cancer." He said nothing, had no words, and for some reason I wanted to take care of him and so I said, "I'll be all right. It's in my breast, they can operate . . . but they have to take the whole thing . . ."

"I'll come over. You'll be okay, Maddy. You're strong. You'll be okay."

He held me. Then we sat in separate chairs in the living room for what seemed like half an hour but was probably only a few minutes. In bed, he held me until he fell asleep.

I had to tell my parents and my friends. Everyone was loving and I had never felt so lonely in my life. I had been chosen to show, for now, how we deal with sudden threats of death. That was the only job I could think up to keep me going.

I waited two weeks for surgery, living in a body I was suddenly afraid of. Michael bought a video recorder and we watched funny movies.

"How are you going to feel about my body when I only have one breast?"

"I don't know." He shrugged. That made me laugh. Michael

did not know how to make up words of comfort and rarely professed to know a thing before he knew it. I loved him for that, more now than ever.

I couldn't eat. Michael coaxed me. I ate a chicken wing for him and one bite of potato. "Some greens," he said. "Come on, Maddy, just a little bit of greens." He was too young to have to live with this.

But Michael loved me.

Afterward, when I looked into the mirror at the neatly drawn pink line across the bony surface where my breast had been, I sometimes cried. After a while, sometimes I'd flex my muscles, posing like an archer—Diana, one-breasted goddess of the hunt. And Michael loved me.

Three years later—two months after we parted—they found cancer in my other breast. Michael still loves me, that's a fact. I love him, and we are not together. The breakup wasn't about breasts; it was time for our relationship to end. But there could not possibly, in anybody's nightmares, have been a worse time to get the big C again than two months after we broke up.

"Luck," the doctor said, "bad luck. You are married, aren't you?"

"No."

Like a wounded dog I mourned the loss of Michael.

I sat close up to the full-length mirror. Close, close, knees up against the glass. I'm leaning in, looking, seeing who is there. "Can we do this, Maddy? Can we take it? Can we handle this, or what?" No answer; it's not an easy question. I had to look into my eyes, behind them, see who was still there. "Yes. I'm sorry, so sorry you have to go through this, Maddy, but we can do it." I do it, lose the other breast, and all goes well except that my body's healing cells, in their confusion, form so much scar tissue that it ruins the reconstructive surgery.

I have two new breasts, almost. The reconstruction has to be done over. The scar tissue turned harder and harder and squeezed the implants, trying to get rid of them. The right one feels like a doorknob and looks like a dented tennis ball. The left one has good shape but is hard. In fact, they're both so hard it's uncomfortable to hug another person. I'm told that next time they'll be soft and perfect. But I need a break. I need to live my life for a while without surgery and anesthesia. The last time I was coming to, cold and hollow, sobbing, I was grateful, believing myself brought back from death.

I sit up close to the mirror now, asking myself what the hell I'm doing with the construction worker from across the street. I hear the foreman with the loud voice calling, "Brendaaaan, Brendaaaan!" I leave the mirror and go to my window and see Brendan, up in the construction.

He called once before he left New Jersey and then again when he reached my corner. We agreed to meet outside my building. I had no intention of having him come up to my apartment, and I wasn't about to let him touch me, no matter how sweet he sounded on the phone. I didn't even know him, and I had no business thinking about anything so personal as touching or cancer or breasts. You couldn't tell a thing about them in my clothes: an electric blue tank top, a jacket, black and Japanese, the slacks from France. And Brendan? I could have placed my mouth, lips apart, over the spot on his neck where his silky ash-brown hair lay freshly cut, but it was our first date. Both of us were shining, buffed and scrubbed.

Sitting next to him in a sporty red car while he drove around the block to a garage, I said, "What are you looking at?" I was feisty, happy, like being on my first date at the age of twelve, only knowing everything I know now. So, "What are you looking at?"

"You. You look terrific."

"Thanks. Whose car is this, anyway?"

"Mine. I have three cars—the truck, a BMW and this Toyota. I love cars. If I weren't in construction I'd be a race car driver."

"Go for it."

"Nah. I'm too old. I'm twenty-five."

I was so much older than he that it didn't matter any more. I was having such a good time that it didn't matter if we never had another date. And it was getting better; Brendan hurrying around my side of the car to open up the door, offering his hand, commandeering a bar stool for me in the crowded restaurant, ordering and handing me my drink. Budweiser was his beer. Like on TV. I'd never been out with anyone who drank Budweiser. I looked up at him standing solicitously by me.

"What did you do before you got into construction?"

"I played professional baseball. Right out of high school. I was scouted and they wanted me—the New York Yankees wanted me."

"No kidding?"

"Yeah. I had to decide what to do. You know, go to college or play ball, but then they offered me a hundred thousand dollars, right out of high school—I wasn't gonna turn it down. And I was good."

"What happened?"

"Couldn't take it. I played in the minors for a year. Too much pressure, too much travel. I don't use drugs, no way, and you wouldn't want to see those guys with the cocaine, all night every night, in the back of the bus. I played two hundred and forty-seven games in two hundred and fifty days . . . Nah, I couldn't take it. Couldn't kiss ass, either, which is what you have to do. Nah, I quit."

"So much for baseball. What about construction?"

"Plenty of money, good hours, different locations. It's good. My uncle is big in the union, my cousin too. Want another drink?"

"Sure."

"If you think construction workers are lowlifes, you should ride on a bus with baseball players from the sticks."

"I never said I think construction workers are lowlifes."

"I know, but you know what I mean. You should hear them comin' into work on Monday morning talkin' about the women they were with on Saturday night—'hey, did you do this, did you do that? I really gave it to her good.' You know what they are? They're male sluts."

"You don't do that?"

"No. I don't even go out with girls. I never had time when I was in baseball and I don't bother with girls now."

"Brendan, come on . . ."

"No, I mean it. I don't. I mean, I met you, you're interesting, a woman, and I like you and we're having a few drinks—it's different. I don't know." His face behind his grin turned a special shade of red again.

"Brendan, do you live at home? With your family, in New Jersey?"

"Yeah. Me and my father bought the house. Why should I pay eight hundred dollars a month for a studio apartment when I can live in a house and give the money to my mother?"

"Who all lives there?"

"Me, my father, my mother, one sister, one brother who's

fourteen, and my baby brother. He's two."

"Omigod."

"Yeah, my folks went to Australia on vacation and got romantic and had an accident. My father's retired on a pension since he had a heart attack—just before my baby brother was born. He fell down on the front lawn. He called for me; I'm his favorite— he's Brendan, too. I'm Brendan Junior. So my mother runs out of the house, she's eight months pregnant, and she jumps on top of him and starts beatin' on his chest and yellin', 'Don't you dare die, goddammit, don't you dare die and leave me here to bring up this kid by myself!' So my father, I swear to God, he survives the attack."

"I love it. What's your mother's name?"

"Bridget . . . It's gettin' noisy in here, hard to talk, you know?"

"You've been doing fine, Brendan, just fine."

"Oh yeah? It's just me . . . Brendan." He laughed and threw his head back, then stopped laughing and looked at me again. I didn't move. I was relaxed, comfortable except for my neck, which had been tilted up because he'd been standing for so long.

"How about we leave here?" he said.

"Sure." I slipped off the stool. I hadn't had too much to drink. I had no plan, I wasn't nervous anymore; in fact, I had no problems. He kept talking as we walked the two blocks to my building and went in.

He was nuts for my apartment, particularly the soft gray leather couch, onto which he draped himself almost upside down. "This is great," he said. "Can I live here?"

"On my couch?"

"Yeah. I like it. Let's go out and get some beer. How's that? Is that okay?"

"Okay."

We went out onto the street, and Brendan took my hand as we walked, holding it as though I were his sweetheart. I love that stuff. I'm stuck there, I guess, in the place where girls feel small and taken care of and all the starch goes out of the resolve to never give yourself up again when a big strong man with good looks and courting manners lifts you up and carries you, or holds your hand. That stuff melts me. And it hasn't always gotten me in trouble. I've had some long good times with men. I can't complain.

"You're sweet," I said.

"So are you."

I didn't disagree; I am sweet and, since my troubles, more easygoing than I used to be.

"After you?" Brendan said, bowing as he held the front door open, under his arm a brown-bagged six-pack of Bud for him, one Watney's Ale for me.

Minutes later, at a distance from me on the enormous curving sofa, sipping beer, his feet stripped down to socks, Brendan was at home.

"Try and relax," I said.

He laughed. "I like it here. It's beautiful."

I thanked him for the compliment. He moved to sit next to me, so close that his thigh rested against mine.

"Brendan," I said, "I don't know how to act. I feel funny. This is my first date in seven years, I mean, since seven years ago . . ."

"Is it?" He was smiling. "I'm just sitting next to you. It's nice."

"Yes, it is."

"You don't have to worry, I don't have to have sex with you. We don't have to have sex, but we could hug. Could we do that?"

I moved away only just enough to face him. "I don't know. I'm scared of having sex ever again, with anybody."

"I've only had sex a few times—with one woman three years ago and then a couple of times since then."

"No."

"Yeah. That's me. I told you, I don't go out much."

"You're telling me the truth, aren't you?"

"Yeah."

Right then and there, I decided he was an angel, honest to God; an Irish, practically-a-virgin angel with a white-light smile beaming at me all these months, sent to me this night—to my own living room.

"Are you real?" I asked him.

"Yeah."

He was. And he was sent because it was my turn for goodies; yes, I remember asking for them, something for Madeleine now, please, goodies, a sign, anything to let me know I will be loved again.

"Were you always an angel—the good boy, the best boy in your family?"

"Yeah, I went to church, went by all the rules. I'm the favorite . . ."

"I know. I even know why. But are you real?"

"Yes, it's just me, Brendan. Can we hug? I'd like to hug. We can hold each other, can't we?"

"There's something I have to tell you. Something about myself . . . about my body."

"What's the matter with your body?"

"Nothing," I said, my hands protecting, pressing the hard implants in my chest. "It's my breasts. They're different. Brendan, I've had breast cancer. Twice."

"My God," he said, "what a strong woman you are. Look what you've been through. My God, you're terrific!"

Was that it? I said "cancer" and he said "terrific"? I held onto my chest and laughed.

"Brendan, are you real?"

"Yeah. So, what're they like? They look okay from here."

"Well, they're hard, and uncomfortable, and they have to be done over."

"Let's see. Can I see them?"

Of course I hesitated, but I never took my eyes off him.

"Yes," I said, lifting up my shirt. "There. See?"

"They're not bad. You shouldn't feel bad about that. Can I touch them?"

"Sure."

The angel to his fingers. He touched them without making a pass at me.

"They're fine," he said. "You're a fine woman."

I pulled down my shirt and picked up my glass of beer. Done. The big-deal issue of the breasts. The tears over Michael's having been the only one to love me in a damaged state. Done.

Horizontal on the long stretch of soft gray leather, we embraced. Sweet sweet sweet sweet angel, was what I thought, Brendan, Irish angel, whose hair smells of sunflower and clover honey.

"So," he said, lifting his head from my shoulder, looking at me nose to nose, "do you kiss?"

"I don't know."

"Come on, let's kiss."

Sweet sweetness, he stopped me all night long, every time I moved in bed, he stopped me from pulling up my camisole.

"Don't. There's nothing wrong with you."

The next morning he went back to New Jersey. The next afternoon he telephoned.

"Do you miss me? I miss you," he said.

"What can I make when I have you to dinner?"

"Steak."

"I don't eat meat."

"Fish sticks, then."

"How about spaghetti?"

"With meat sauce?"

"No."

"With meat balls?"

I laughed. "I told you, I don't eat meat."

He laughed. "I can't make it anyway. I gotta coach my brother's high school team."

"Yes, my angel. I'll see you . . . in the neighborhood."

"Okay, that's okay, Madeleine. You're a real fine woman."

Where's this going to get you, Maddy? Take the gift and go. Say thank you, thank the sweet man and go.

"Brendaaaan, Brendaaaan!" I'd hear outside my window and I'd know he was at work high up in construction.

To My Uterus

APRIL LINDNER

Because I cannot see you, they say I will not miss you.
Because I cannot touch you, not feel your churning distinct
from my body's daily making of marrow, blood and
spit, they say I do not need you.
Because you speak to me only in contractions, in bloating of
breasts and belly and
Because I should not miss the gaudy flag that you unfurl
each month, announcing you are empty, they say I am
well rid of you.
Because I can adopt or choose to mother books of poems, they
say that I am wise to let them take you.
Because I cannot see you, I must trust these men who spread
latex fingers in me, bump against you, say your rosy
sides are mottled.

I cannot see you and they say cancer runs its small hard
hands along your pink flesh, claiming you.
I cannot see you and they say you will harden, clot, and still
the cancer will not stop.
I cannot see you and they say you will betray me to your
captor.

Soon, they say, I will see you for what you are: plush purse
filled with death.
Soon, they say, I will learn to live one stone lighter.
Soon, they say, I will learn to walk without your weight
pressing me to earth.
Soon, they say, I will learn to love again the love that lasts
for hours till his eyes and mine are crusted shut
with sleep, until the sheets are twisted and sticky,
half thrown to the floor.
Soon I will love again the delicate tilting of my pelvis
against his, the clasping and unclasping.
Soon I will love again the search, blind reaching for
rebirth, for you, the sources, for you, pulsating star
that men have always coveted.

168

Breasts

SANDY POLISHUK

Breasts make the difference between a girl and a woman. Having grown breasts means you have grown up. I really believed that. It surprised me later when I heard menstruation treated as the rite of passage into womanhood. For me, it was always breasts.

As a little girl, I was nearly obsessed with the desire to know what my breasts would be like when they arrived. I would lie in my bed and solemnly, silently pray to see a sixteen-year-old me in my dreams.

The first girl in my class to develop breasts was Judy Channing. That was in the sixth grade. Judy would wear thin, snug sweaters, no bra. I was outraged. I was jealous. I was flat.

I began to notice swelling nipples under the sweaters of other girls at school. Finally, my own change began. I begged my mother for a brassiere. It was important to have its shadow showing under one's blouse, to have a pair of straps on one's shoulders. At last it was permitted. My bra looked more like a garter belt than a brassiere, but I didn't mind.

I draped myself on the couch and proudly let my sweatshirt slip to the side at the neckline so that the shoulder strap of my bra was exposed. Nan, my friend whose breasts were *really* there, was shocked. "Do you have a bra already? My mom thinks they don't make bras small enough for me, but if you have one . . ." I had the advantage of an older sister, who'd started with a AAA.

Eventually, I could fill a brassiere. I had all kinds: underwire, strapless, longline, even a "merry widow" with its bones which dug into my too-high hips.

I started wearing a bra about two years before I started smoking and got contact lenses. I gave up smoking at twenty-four when I had my first baby, my contacts with my third child (they were too much trouble) at twenty-eight, and my bra when I weaned him a few months later. The smoking, the contact lenses, and the bra are all linked in my memory, relics of my teenage growing-up years.

It was in the late 1960s, and bralessness was a symbol of

freedom and rebellion. My mother objected. She said my breasts would sag when I got older. I said I could wear a bra then if they did. What she really objected to, I think, was the sensuality of my unharnessed breasts.

One member of my women's consciousness-raising group said, "You have to pass the pencil test. You put a pencil under your breast, and if it falls, you don't need a bra." I ignored the test. I was more interested in comfort than appearances.

Already I had given up girdles, and now I gave up razors, makeup, high heels, and skirts. I didn't have to dress for a job. My husband was supporting me. My style was alternative, bohemian, casual, ethnic—no fitted blouses or jackets with darts which might have demanded a bra for a decent fit. When I stopped censoring my wardrobe, I worried what some people might think when they noticed my bralessness, but eventually I stopped thinking about it.

As I lay naked in my bed reading one warm evening nearly twenty years later, I brushed my hand against my left breast. I felt a marble-like lump under my skin. It proved to be cancer.

I agonized over the decision to give up my breast. My breast for my life—obviously a rational trade. But my attachment to my breast was deeper than rationality. I loved my breast, enjoyed it, wanted it.

I stood in front of the mirror trying to push my breast out of the way, trying to see what my chest would look like without it. I couldn't imagine it. I wanted to find a woman who had undergone a mastectomy, wanted to ask her to show me, to let me touch her where her breast had been.

I walked around looking for one-breasted women, knowing they were there, thousands of them, more every year, and yet I couldn't find them. They were hiding behind protheses and reconstruction.

How odd. How odd the whole idea seemed to me, right from the beginning. I couldn't understand why someone would want a numb bump on her chest, a thing that is not her but is attached to her, even under her own skin. I could not and still cannot understand. Yet, indeed, many want it.

I longed to shout at those women, "Take off your prostheses! Let the world know! Let us see each other! Let us know each other and demand a halt to this disease!"

I felt very angry. Angry that one-breasted women hide. Angry that breasts have such a distorted importance in our culture that so many of us feel we must pretend we still have them. Angry that this pretense kept me from finding my sisters. Angry that we are lulled into a false complacency because the monstrous number of one-breasted or even un-breasted women is concealed. Angry that my one-breastedness would be seen as an oddity when I knew it was, in fact, all too common.

I had rarely examined my breasts. There were all sorts of lumps and bumps in there. I had always thought I wouldn't be able to recognize a cancerous lump. Why wasn't I told how different this would feel? Why wasn't mammography included in my medical coverage? Why had I been ignorant of the correlation between the amount of fat in a country's diet and its breast cancer rate?

I watched in admiration as people with AIDS and their supporters organized for research, for treatment, for release of drugs, for services. I wondered why cancer victims are so silent, separate, and hiding.

The night before entering the hospital for my mastectomy, my lover, Alex, and I went to a movie. We decided to see "Steaming," because we'd heard it was funny. The film was set in a women's steam bath. If I had thought about it, I would have realized that this film would be full of naked women, women with big, beautiful, double-breasted chests. The entire time I was watching the movie I was aware they all had two breasts. We *don't* all have two breasts. I know that now. But in "Steaming" they all did. When we left the film, I said to Alex, "I wish they'd had some one-breasted women," and then I cried, standing on the sidewalk. I cried bitterly.

That night I had the first dream I remembered since I found the lump. I am at the ticket window in a European train station trying to reserve a seat, but they are all gone. The woman behind the wrought iron window goes out of her way to be helpful and finds me one. I am very grateful and like her so much. I start to leave the window but glance back. She isn't wearing a shirt. She has three breasts, horizontally across her chest. The breast on the far right is larger than the others. My dream self thinks, "Oh, not everyone has two!"

Many of my friends were wearing brassieres again. Standards had changed, and those with larger breasts found bralessness uncomfortable or ungainly now. But my breasts were fairly small and didn't sag as predicted. Unlike many women who think their breasts are too small or too large or too something, I had always liked mine. They were fine. I felt comfortable and attractive braless. I liked to wear snug tank tops, the kind that wouldn't work with a bra. I liked the freedom from straps that dig and slip.

The idea of starting to wear a bra in order to keep a prosthesis in place was too ridiculous. If I didn't wear a bra when I had two breasts, it didn't make sense to wear a bra with one. I made up my mind to face the world as I would be—one-breasted—but I worried about how people would react. Would women who did wear prostheses be angry at me, criticize me?

I would now be an amputee, a freak, different, looked at strangely. Maybe I would be treated differently. A blind woman once told me that people treated her as if she were stupid. I had had years of inhaling the belief that the ugly, the abnormal, the less than perfect should be hidden. I remember sitting with my family in a car while a very large woman walked by wearing snug pants. "Doesn't she have any shame?" my mother said. In her day, even pregnant women hid. And breasts have a sexual connotation; "nice" women don't display them too boldly or talk about them in mixed company.

I found myself identifying with people who have awful scars, mutilations, or cerebral palsy, people who are obviously disabled, people whom my mother might feel should have more shame than to let themselves be seen. I began to wonder how it is for those people facing the world.

In another dream, I am with a blind woman. We talk about her being blind. She is extraordinarily well adjusted and competent. In fact, she is simultaneously reading and driving a car. Somehow I would make the world know I still had all my powers.

I had seen Audre Lorde read her poetry a few years earlier. How shocked I was when she first stood up! I had not known about her mastectomy. Here was a large woman with one big breast and one flat side, wearing a turtleneck T-shirt. It was so obvious. I was horrified. But I sat and looked at her as she read. In the hour my shock and horror had passed, and I admired her courage, and I thought I understood.

Almost the first thing I did after the doctor called to say it was bad news was to buy Lorde's *The Cancer Journals*. That night I couldn't sleep. I got up at 2:00 in the morning and read the book, paying special attention to the chapter on prostheses. I thought: thank God someone is out there who agrees with me, who understands.

I, too, refuse to be ashamed that I have had cancer. I refuse to be ashamed that I have had a mastectomy. My self-worth is not diminished. I will not act as if I have something to hide. I will not pretend to have a breast that I don't have.

I silently cheered when a woman in my breast cancer support group, who had had a double mastectomy and wore no prosthesis, exclaimed, "All of them—the doctors, the Reach to Recovery women, the books—they all say, 'Here's your choice: reconstruction or prosthesis.' There's no one out there saying, 'You don't have to do anything.'"

Everything I heard in the group confirmed my decision. All but one woman disliked their prostheses, complaining of discomfort, slipping, and chafing. Jill Ireland wrote that the prosthesis is for those who look at her.[1] It allows them to forget what has happened; for her, the prosthesis is the opposite—it's a constant reminder.

The day after the last drain tube from my surgery was removed, I awakened to discover fluid had accumulated and was sloshing under my skin. A little mini-breast growing again. It fed all my fantasies. My friend Mary has lost an eye. She said, "Wouldn't it be nice if we were like crabs? I could grow a new eye, and you could grow a new breast." Yes, wouldn't it.

The doctors would be glad to give me a new breast. All I have ever had to do is ask and endure more surgery. But the very idea of a thing attached to me is distasteful. And it would not look or feel or act like my own breast; it wouldn't fool me, and I am the one I want to fool. It wouldn't have feeling. I would have to wear a bra to look matched, like the woman in my support group who said, "I'm a pert sixteen-year-old on one side and a sagging fifty-nine-year-old on the other."

I care most how I look to myself, how I look naked, how I feel to *my* touch. I have come back to the thought of reconstruction any number of times, but it is only a fantasy, not unlike the fantasy of my breast growing back. So the answer is always the same: no, not for me.

Just home from the hospital, I had another dream. My grandfather is cuddling me, and his hand brushes upon the empty place. Quickly, he moves it to the other side. I say, "It's all right, it's quite numb, really. Go ahead, touch me there." Then he is feeling my chest, and I am saying, "See, there's the muscle, and there are the ribs. It's just gone, like a boy." It was time for Alex to touch my new body, for both of us to begin the process of getting used to the change.

I hadn't thought about the mastectomy when I took my first bath after my surgery. I had spent so much time in the bathtub, time learning to love my body, learning to appreciate its beauty from that vantage point of looking down past my breasts to my belly and thighs. But sitting in the bathtub, I felt the shock of the breast not being there. Instead, there was this terrible bony flatness and the bright scar. It was different from standing and looking in the mirror, different from looking down when I was sitting up. I was not prepared for the difference I saw while stretched out in a tub. I felt a tremendous sadness.

Three years have passed, but I am still sometimes surprised when I see myself naked in the mirror. I will go to the sink to brush my teeth and be jolted by the absence, the deformity. I am continually amazed that Alex has come to terms with my new body so well. He misses my breast, too, but he still finds me sexy.

I know I have to get used to the changes in my body in order to go on with my life, to not be destroyed emotionally by cancer and mastectomy. And sometimes I even like my new chest. I can understand what other women are saying when they talk about being a boy on one side. Especially clothed, my chest often looks okay to me, kind of clean and neat and young.

But I don't think I will ever be completely used to the idea. My breast has been lopped off! Amputated. My beautiful, lovely, sensitive breast, cut up in a laboratory. Looked at and analyzed by quadrants. Described in a pathology report as "a left breast with an erect nipple."

Mastectomy is an experience so common, more common every day. In Oregon alone, at least twenty-five women have mastectomies every week.[2] Thousands of breasts have been taken. Will any of us forget that we once had two? Will we ever get over the loss completely? Should anyone—should a society—accept this mutilation? I have to accept the new contour of my chest in order to continue as a functioning and healthy person. At the same time, I refuse to accept the status quo. It is unacceptable for over eleven percent of us to suffer this disease.

I felt naked my first time out as a one-breasted woman, even though I wore a thick hand-woven Guatemalan huipil shirt that completely hid the contours of my chest.

My surgery was in early October. I told Alex that I wanted to go to the Halloween Ball dressed as an Amazon, a one-breasted warrior. At first he laughed, but when he realized I was serious, he became upset. At the time, the idea seemed to me to be a good way to tell people, tell them I'm all right. Tell them I'm not ashamed; they don't have to avoid me. He said it was too much; it would make people too uncomfortable. The point became moot. I wasn't well enough to go.

Then, only weeks after I lost my breast, I began to lose my hair to chemotherapy. My beautiful hair, my best feature. This loss, coming so soon after the loss of my breast, was shattering. I had already come to hate telling people what was going on. They got too upset. It was hard enough taking care of myself; I didn't want to have to take care of them, too. I wanted them to already know when I saw them, or else I didn't want to be forced to tell them just because of my baldness.

I went to a performance feeling quite chic, an exotic scarf with a beautiful silver pin covering my nearly bald head. Then, standing in the gallery waiting to be seated, I saw a man with hair like mine. I wanted us to acknowledge each other, at least to make eye contact, but I was hiding. He didn't know me as I knew him. I stopped hiding my baldness, too.

My color improved and my hair grew back when I finished chemotherapy, but I still hated the reaction to my revelation of cancer. So I usually said nothing and worried instead that people would notice my breast is missing. And then they would realize: this means cancer.

Cancer—the "C" word. It took me three years to understand that I can tell people I have had cancer without freaking them out. It's different now than it was when I told people that I was under treatment for cancer. When one says, "I have cancer," many people hear, "I am dying." But now they can look at me and see a healthy, active person.

I feel a need to broach the subject in order—I think—to put others at ease. But sometimes I wonder if other people are even bothered by my one-breastedness. I wonder if they even notice it. Maybe my need to talk about cancer is only for my own sake, to put *myself* at ease.

I am most comfortable in the company of people who already know, people with whom it is all right for me to refer in passing to cancer or chemotherapy, people with whom I don't have to wonder if they are noticing my asymmetrical chest. Then I can forget about it. I don't remember my previous consciousness, but I suspect I now overrate the breast's visual importance. My friends keep telling me that my one-breastedness is not noticeable, but I find it hard to believe them. *I* look at other people's bodies. *I* notice breasts. Did I before I lost one? And then there are the times when I know that other people see. I was at a resort with a communal hot tub and sauna. No one, except for one small child, wore a bathing suit. I gritted my teeth and took my clothes off. I entered the sauna alone. There were two other women there. In a few moments they got up and left. Did they leave because they were ready to or because of their discomfort with my mastectomy?

Later, Alex and I sat in the hot tub submerged to our collarbones, the churning water obscuring the rest of our bodies. A couple joined us. We had a long and enjoyable conversation. The woman had a broken arm and carefully held the cast out of the water. We talked about her arm easily. Then it was time to get out of the tub. I stood and exposed my body. Nothing was said.

I took a scuba course. For a week I spent most of the day with the same small group of men. I wore a tank suit, and nothing was hidden. And nothing was said.

Children frequently ask Mary, "What happened to your eye?" But even children seem to know not to inquire about a breast. It is hard for me to expose my maimed body, but the silence is even more uncomfortable, a wall of isolation encircling me. I want to lose my self-consciousness, to go on, to buy and wear clothes without first thinking: how revealing is this shirt? Is this material too thin and clinging?

It is only now, three years after my surgery, that I see myself passing into the stage of being able to wear an ordinary T-shirt in public comfortably. It is only now that I have realized that the past three years have been a transition period somewhat like my former transition periods of budding nipples and then the shedding of my bra.

In a dream I am holding my child. She is angry and upset. She is a tiny thing with one little eye. Her head falls out of its socket, like a toy. For a time, a second eye appears on her head. I worry that she isn't going to make it, but she starts getting better.

NOTES

1. Ireland, Jill, *Life Wish*, Little, Brown & Co., Boston, 1987, p. 240.

2. There were an estimated 1,700 new breast cancer cases in Oregon in 1989, according to *Cancer Statistics*, American Cancer Society, Atlanta, 1989, page 12. In a conversation with me on June 18, 1990, Dr. Andrew G. Glass, an oncologist with Kaiser Permanente in Portland, Oregon, stated that approximately 80 percent of those cases undergo mastectomies; those figures work out to a weekly average of twenty-six mastectomies.

The Swimmer

ROSYLIN DEAN
with assistance from Siobhán Dugan

I felt weird as I watched myself fidget with foam cups and bathing suit straps. In front of the mirror, I pushed at myself this way and that so both breasts would match. When I was a teenager, I wore falsies in my bathing suit because I was very small-breasted. In fact, when I was a teenager, I wore falsies all the time.

I stopped wearing the falsies when I got older, but after the mastectomy I found myself trying to put falsies in my bathing suit again. I couldn't use the regular prosthesis in my bathing suit because that silicone breast provided by the insurance company might get waterlogged, and bathing suits which are specifically designed to deal with this problem are absurdly expensive. Finally, out of exasperation and annoyance, I ended up throwing my foam rubber falsie aside, and now I don't wear anything.

These days when I do my swimming, I wear a tank suit. I'm flat on one side and just flatter on the other. The fact that I am small-breasted really makes it easier. If I were large-breasted on one side and flat on the other, I surely would feel more awkward. I find I am annoyed that I allowed myself, if only briefly, to be caught up in this cultural decree again, reliving a fifteen-year-old's evaluation of herself and her human worth as based on her tit size. In any case, the déjà vu, along with the piles of literature about breast protheses I've collected, caused me to begin thinking about our cult of the breast.

I have recently come across so many versions of this fantasy, this measure of a woman's worth by the size of her breasts. Always there is the memory of myself standing in front of my mirror. There is my friend Sandy, whose family yelled at her when they heard the diagnosis, as though she were bringing them dishonor. There was Maria, whose husband forbade her to have her cancerous breast removed. She died for her obedience, a martyr to the mythical primacy of the breast.

I first heard Maria's story when I returned to work after my chemotherapy with my half-plucked look hooded under knit caps.

Maria's daughter Karen is a co-worker of mine, and she took me in hand. She'd had some beautician's training, and for several months she spent her lunch hours caressing and nursing my hair back to decency. "I'm doing this for you," Karen told me, "and for my mother. She died of cancer, and I couldn't do anything for her." Maria had called her daughter one day, crying because she was worried that her husband would be unable to handle the situation. She didn't think about whether she would live or die; she thought about how *he* would feel if she were a "mutilated" woman. And then he did forbid her to have her breast removed, and she died. "Sometimes when I comb your hair," Karen said, "I imagine it's hers, and that we are talking about her recovery."

Our cultural worship of the breast—ultimately responsible for Maria's death—isn't just a marginal or isolated attitude. The eminence of the breast is institutionalized; even the insurance companies and the state are in on it. My co-worker, Debbie, needed extensive cancer surgery on her face. Her eye was removed, along with her palate and the top of her mouth—all cut away. Her teeth were removed, and her cheekbone had to be reconstructed. She was forced to fight her insurance company to get them to pay for the palate. And how could she function without that? After the operation, Debbie was sent by her doctor to a specialist for a palate prosthesis. But the specialist was not on her insurance company's approved physicians list, and they refused to pay. She and her doctor followed an appeals procedure, and after much arguing the insurance company agreed to pay 50 percent of the cost. They claimed that her dental insurance should be held responsible, while the dental insurance claimed otherwise. Debbie's eye surgeon spoke to the insurance company about an eye replacement and was told that such a procedure was merely cosmetic and they would not cover it. Debbie was also told that if the prosthesis had been a breast it would have been completely covered. She still doesn't have an artificial eye; she wears a patch.

I don't understand. I know that losing a breast is psychologically damaging. But losing an eye is not? Women who are victims of breast cancer and lose a breast should be able to have reconstructive surgery if they wish it. But when breasts are worth paying for and an eye isn't, something is wrong.

It isn't just the insurance companies at the bottom of this lopsided injustice. The State Insurance Code issues the mandates under which insurance companies operate, and those codes include specific kinds of coverage as well as general guidelines. Breast reconstructive surgery or breast prostheses are covered by state mandate. Why aren't other parts of the body—like eyes—also covered? Why has the breast been singled out? Strong lobbies have pushed through the coverage of breast replacements. Perhaps the fact that so many women now are breast cancer victims is a part of the reason for insurance coverage of breast reconstruction. Or is this attention coming from the cult-like worship of the breast? Perhaps it's a bit of both. The only thing we can know for sure is that real regard for the lives of women has never played a part in determining the rules of the insurance game.

Our women's bodies are objects in this culture, objects which have become alien even to ourselves. I went to a conference on breast cancer one weekend where one of the speakers dramatized the prohibitions that come with that objectification. She walked onto the stage clutching her breasts. "See," she said, "it's okay to touch yourself. It's okay! I'm right up here on the stage doing it, and you can do it, too." She then did an informal survey of the women in the audience to see how many women did monthly breast self-examinations. Most women raised their hands, but some women did not. These women were at least conscious enough of the dangers of breast cancer to be at this conference, but even among these women there were some who don't "touch" themselves. I can't help but wonder how many of the 43,000 women who will die from breast cancer this year would have been spared if this were not a culture of breast worship in which so many of us just don't feel right about touching these awesome objects, our own breasts.

I wonder about myself and the world and the people around me. I know how fragile life is. That fragility has become very personal. Just so has my anger become much keener, my anger at the misuse of power which affects the daily lives of people, and even kills them—the power of a doctor over the patient, the power of a government over the people, the power of one country over a weaker one, the power of sexual objectification over the quality of human life.

Headwrap

NOELLE CASKEY

This is a story about transcendence. It's also a story about loss, grief, rage, nausea and fear. It's the story of what I gained when I lost my hair.

Oh, what an awful world I had entered when I found myself waiting to be evaluated by the Tumor Board at the Stanford Medical Center. Alone in the examining room, where I would shortly be poked, prodded and interrogated, I found nothing to occupy me but some copies of *Cope* magazine, a publication for cancer patients and their families.

I found stories of women who had discovered breast cancer during the last trimester of pregnancy and had been forced to decide whether to risk the baby by having chemo or risk themselves by waiting until after the birth. I found other stories I couldn't read or look at. What held me with a perverse fascination were the stories of Hollywood models who had determinedly kept themselves beautiful with scarves and makeup tricks while their hair and eyelashes fell out.

That was where I drew the line. I had already accepted in principle the mastectomy my then surgeon had recommended, but somehow that was different from the public disfigurement of going bald. I knew I couldn't face it. If I had to have chemotherapy I would stay at home with the curtains drawn and would never go out or see anyone until it was over. I was no Hollywood model, skilled at the paraphernalia of personal appearance and the art of self-presentation. I was just a shy, ordinary woman without the least interest in glamour. No way would I become one of those upbeat, happy cancer patients depicted in that awful magazine. When the news came back that my lymph nodes were okay, my relief was not so much about the increased odds for survival the results gave me, but more because I would be spared the ordeal of hair loss.

By the time I had learned that four out of four oncologists recommended chemotherapy for me, I had already come a long way in accepting the cancer patient identity I had been so desperate to refuse that day at Stanford. The daily discipline of radiation treatments was responsible for this shift. Sitting in the radiation oncology waiting room day after day with other cancer patients made it impossible for me to think of myself as someone who had only had surgery; instead, I continued to be a cancer patient among other cancer patients, some of whose stories I came to learn.

Indeed, when the news was handed down to me that chemotherapy was in store for me, I was grateful for the company and support of those other patients, especially a trio of ladies I had come to think of as "the brain tumors." Each day I sat with them hearing their catalogue of symptoms ("I had trouble with nouns. Did you have trouble with nouns? I could never remember the word 'chiropractor,' and I always had to say 'acupuncturist.'") and noting the variety of head coverings they used to conceal the scars and baldness that come with brain surgery. One had a friend who designed and sold turbans which she marketed to chemotherapy patients. I asked for a color sample and address, happy at having a possible solution come to me without my having to seek it out.

The turbans, though convenient, seemed to call attention to their wearers, and I was not sure I wanted to spend however long my treatment took looking like a little round-headed doll. All the books counseled solving the problem of hair loss before it arose, so I spent some time with the telephone book, trying to figure out who sold wigs and where I could get one.

Buying a wig turned out to be not such an easy proposition, hampered as I was by my shyness concerning my personal appearance and my reluctance to confess to total strangers what was happening to me. My husband and I located the name and address of a San Francisco wig supplier and went early one day before my radiation to see what sort of solution we could find there. The address led me to a faceless warren of a building full of all sorts of obscure businesses. Diligently we tracked the wig supplier to his lair on the second floor, tiptoeing nervously around seemingly endless corners before we found a door with the right label. Instead of an anonymous display of wigs, we saw only a round, bald little man sitting at a desk, writing. We peered in at him, then fled shivering while he pursued us down the hall like a Dickensian wraith, crying desperately after us, "Can I help you? Can I help you?" No, it just wasn't possible.

Our next effort in the wig department followed my first treatment. My husband's parents had come to town to lend support to both of us, and when I had recovered a little from the trauma of that first devastatingly messy experience, my husband, my mother-in-law, and I hit the downtown department stores in search of a wig. The crucial player in this search was my mother-in-law. Where I am shy, she is bold; where I am retiring, she is demanding; where I flee before the proud looks of saleswomen, she has no hesitation in exacting service.

Even my mother-in-law, however, could not create wigs where there were none. Not until our third department store did we find a wig department which had more than a few falls and switches for elegant ladies getting ready for evening and the opera. We pulled open drawer after drawer and had pulled out piles of boxes before a young woman could interest herself in helping us. In spite of her lack of enthusiasm (and my mother-in-law's predilection for selecting wigs that matched her hair instead of mine) we were finally successful in locating a specimen that approximated my own shade of brown mixed with gray.

In triumph, we returned to the city hotel room where my husband's parents were staying in order to display our find. My father-in-law promptly seized our purchase and draped it over his balding head so that it covered one eye and the tag dangled ridiculously in front of his face. He looked like Harpo Marx. Somehow that act of his underlined for me the futility of the enterprise. Wearing that wig I did not look like myself but rather like some caricature of myself, or someone else's idea of what a woman should be. The artificial hair mounded over my head and made me feel like a laughable stranger. I was glad to have the wig, but I could not wear it.

My hair didn't fall out immediately, but it didn't wait for my second treatment, either. My first warning of what was to come (although I didn't understand what it meant at the time) was a feeling that my scalp was unbearably hot and itchy. Over the next few nights more and more hair collected on my pillow, so that when I woke up the pillow was covered by a miniature forest of hair. The typical chemotherapy hair loss scenario is to find gobs of hair swirling down the drain in the shower, but it didn't happen that way for me. There was just a steady attrition which gradually left me looking more and more patchy.

When my hair started falling out, all the things about which I had been so frightened that day in the Stanford Oncology Clinic became my realities. Somehow I had to learn to cope, inadequate as I felt myself to the task. I had long since understood that my illusion about cancer patients absenting themselves from the daily world during the course of their treatments was just that—an illusion. It was not possible or even desirable for me to stay at home with the shades drawn for the entire six months I was scheduled for chemotherapy. I had to do something else.

It helped more than I can say, of course, to have met the "brain tumors" and heard their stories and seen their ways of meeting the shaved heads and jagged scars that went with their disease. I sent for one of their friend's turbans, though I instinctively disliked the flat look which it gave to my head. I couldn't feel like myself; the change was too marked, too obvious, too declaratory of my new status as a fearsome cultural object, taboo, woman without hair, cancer patient.

I tried hats. I had one straw hat with a sewn-in scarf that wrapped and tied around my throat. I don't know if I chose black deliberately or whether it was the only color they had when I bought it, but one day in that hat was enough. It felt peculiar to wear a hat indoors, and the scarf part wrapped my ears as well so that it was hard to hear what people were saying. I already felt cut off by what was happening to me; the black hat made it worse.

At first, I could manage by tying a scarf flapper-style around my head to cover the worst patches, but as the hair loss became more thorough and acute, I could no longer let anything show, both because of the way it would look and also because I risked sunburning my scalp. How unfamiliar my head became! I was unprepared for the slightly greasy feeling of a naked scalp (I now understood the shine gleaming from the heads of bald men), and I began to experience my head differently, as though it were a giant muscle at the top of my neck rather than an entirely separate part of my body.

It was not only my head hair which I lost. My pubic hair was also falling out in a disconcerting reversal of puberty. I remembered how deformed I had felt when I first developed pubic hair, as though the purity of my body was being violated by a gross excrescence. How surprised I was to find that the curved shape of my pubis had remained the same during all those intervening years, that nothing had changed underneath the growth of maturity.

The only difference between my body and that of a baby girl was its size. I was not sure how I felt about the discovery of this underlying continuity; it seemed too much like a regression, a going backwards, to be entirely comfortable.

It's not possible to lose your hair without experiencing depression and anxiety. I don't know what the symbolic value of hair is, but that it has some deep meaning is clear from the stories of women having their heads shaved as punishment for consorting with the enemy or as preparation for entering the convent. One time I was experimenting with one of my scarves and a remaining lock of hair got caught in its folds. I pulled, attempting to free the hair from the scarf; instead, my hair came off in my hand. For minutes afterwards I trembled, my heart pounding.

A few days after my second treatment, my friend Ruth had a mastectomy. The drama of her diagnosis and surgery had unfolded as my life in the radiation oncology waiting room was drawing to a close; the fact that I had been through the experience myself made her cancer both harder and easier to bear. The morning of her surgery, she called me over to her hospital room because there was no one else to whom she could entrust her pearl earrings. She unfastened them from her own ears and put them on my ears. Small though they were, those beautiful pearls of Ruth's did more than anything to reconcile me to my life without hair. By then I knew that some form of headwrap would be necessary for me from then on. As awkward, uncomfortable and unready as I felt, the pearls shining in my earlobes made me feel protected, as though they outshone all my deficiencies.

This is not to say that suddenly the difficulty of coping with hair loss disappeared. No, indeed. I remember all too clearly an uncomfortable evening at one of San Francisco's most elegant restaurants, where we had gone to celebrate the birthday of a close friend. I had made the mistake of trying a chiffon scarf as a headwrap; it was hot and slippery and kept coming untied so that I spent the evening in an agony of miserable self-consciousness worthy of the worst nightmares of adolescence.

I did finally learn that cotton was the only fabric which would work, and I learned a way of tying cotton scarves around my head so that they stayed put. Once doing this had become routine, it was easier to go out in the world than I had anticipated. I would dress in the morning and stand in front of the mirror and make a grimace at myself, then wrap, twist, and knot until I was ready.

Sometimes I would think, "This isn't so bad"; at other times, "This is awful." Familiarity bred both comfort and resentment. But I coped.

I enjoyed particularly the encounters with young women who were too inexperienced to understand what was happening to me. "Oh, I love the way you tie your scarf!" they would coo at me from behind the counters of stores or as they took an order in a restaurant. "Could you show me how to do it?" It pleased me to think that not everyone identified me as a cancer patient, that for some my odd garb was a plus, not a minus.

Headwrap opened another world to me as well, one that I had not anticipated. Even in a city as cosmopolitan as Berkeley, few other women appear in public with heads elaborately wrapped and tied in fabric, and those who do are often women of color. Suddenly I became like one of them. Black women whose beautiful headdresses made me want to applaud would smile and salute me as though we shared some secret. I was pleased and puzzled to find myself in this new sisterhood; when I learned later that voodoo priestesses cover the crowns of their heads with fabric during ceremonies to keep evil spirits from entering, I understood more of this recognition and was pleased.

By the time a month had passed from the beginning of my hair loss, I had for all purposes adapted. I still stood in the shower with both hands clutched to my head to keep more hair from melting away as the water ran over me, but I dressed every morning and went out the door instead of staying at home with the curtains drawn. I went hiking at Mount Rainier. I conducted a poetry reading. I applied for a job, thinking, "I don't need hair to do this," and was accepted. I learned to mark the intimacy and acceptance of my friends by appearing in front of them as I was, without concealment. My mother sent me a picture of myself as a baby, smiling happily with almost no hair. I even posed for a photograph with my balding friend Guido, about whom my mother said, "Always stand next to him and you'll look like you have *lots* of hair!" When the nurse in the oncology ward drew the curtain around me so that I could remove my scarf in privacy before a treatment, I wondered why she bothered. In that setting especially I was comfortable exactly as I was.

From my new perspective I would sometimes glance at a woman passing on the street who had a glorious abundance of hair and think there was something distorted about the way she looked:

"She has too much hair." I had hoped to find that having faced this most feared of experiences, I would never be afraid again. That this is not the case I learned on a swaying suspension bridge over a river chasm at Mount Rainier; and when I sat down in the dentist's chair, the sensation of being tortured did not lessen, although I brought to it a new sense of proportion. And I did learn a new confidence from having been through what many people consider the worst fate which can befall them and from having come to terms with it in my own way. My terrified refusal of the cancer patient identity during my morning at the Stanford Tumor Board had been transformed not just into acceptance, but also into pride and a new belief in what I was capable of.

Of course, having put myself so firmly into headwrap, I had to struggle to come out. My hair started growing back before I had finished my treatments; friends who saw me without my scarf persuaded me that it was time to come out of hiding. Bravely I took myself off to see Joseph, who had played wonderful asymmetric games with my mop of curls in the days when I had them and whom I had avoided during the course of my treatment. I walked into his San Francisco salon looking as though I had been dragged backward through a bush, the new hair uneven and the old still hanging in ragged threads.

Joseph looked at me. "What happened to your hair?" he asked.

"It fell out," I said.

"How come?"

"Chemotherapy."

"What do you want me to do about it?"

"Make me look less like I stuck my finger in the light bulb socket."

"Are you okay now?"

"Yes."

While I was in the changing room, I overheard him telling his co-workers, "She had cancer, but they got it." Then I emerged in my smock and he took up his scissors and made me look like Joan of Arc. Two days later a man I knew slightly passed me on the street and called out, "Wonderful haircut!" as I walked by. That was it. I was out.

Life has gone on since then, but in many ways I am still in the cancer ward, as though having entered, I am destined to remain there. Friends and family members are no more immune than I was to disease. Too often I hear of someone else of my acquaintance newly diagnosed, and Joseph—dear, funny, wonderful Joseph—died of AIDS a few short months after his thirtieth birthday. My response to these tragedies is complicated. Their terribleness is without question, and yet—having been there myself—I believe that something good can grow in the midst of pain, terror and anguish. My friend Lisel said to me, "Watching you go through this made me understand that having cancer isn't about dying; it's about living." The resolve I made on my first chaotic night after diagnosis, to live as long as I am alive, is with me still. I wish nothing better for my friends, be they well or ill.

I still have my headwraps. They sit in a basket next to my dresser, and from time to time I pull them out and look at them. I had thought I might continue to wear them after my hair grew out, but they don't wrap so well over my abundant curls. And, to be honest, the smell of the cloth turns my stomach a bit because it brings back memories of the chemo ward. Once in a while, though, I take one and wrap it around my waist as a sash and go off to work with this private reminder of where I'm going and where I've been.

One-Sided

BARBARA HOFFMAN

In Answer to Audre Lorde's
"Breast Cancer: Power vs. Prosthesis"

She said
if I had courage
I would
be half-flat
half-round

I would honor
the wound
against symmetry

I wouldn't hide
the flat scar
under a silicone breast
placed in my bra

I might as well
open my naked legs
for all
to see
the pink and brown
folds that
hood
my secret self.

Post Diagnosis

SANDRA STEINGRABER

I'm not trying to say it's not
   a good place. It is—
this house where I eat and breathe
and stomp off the cold.
The afternoon sun slants through
a prism I hung on the curtain rod,
scattering clean colors.
I scrub the stout-legged bathtub
to squeakiness, unload
the heavy sacks of groceries.
My green-fibered plants grow
succulent on their window ledges.
I do too.

But sometimes late at night
I hear sounds through my books,
the scruffling of feet
in the walls. I strain to hear
the twitching whiskers . . .
My husband laughs. "Those are pigeons,
San, not rats in the roof."
I dumbly nod and go to bed,
go to warm arms, but protected
against and fearing the contamination of sperm.

I'm not trying to say it's not a good place
but two years after and still
I fear infestation—
staring at specks of dust
that flicker in a spot of sun, shuddering
to think what we breathe into our spongy lungs.
This is absurd, I know.
I look up the word REMISSION
("Release, as from a debt;
restored to an original condition; put back")
and in the kitchen I pour macaroni

into boiling water . . . tiny beetles
spill out with the noodles, swirl
in the pan, belly up, legs curled.

Look, that meant nothing.
I am restored, put back.
I am not like those others,
full of metastases, who are returned
to their lives as guests.
The ones who have no place at all,
who have only a journey
who are packing their bags,
who are leaving now.

A week ago my surgeon rose
from his instruments and laughed—
"Sandra, let's grow old together."
The test's negative. He is a young man
and I told him this was a good place,
a good place to live. But at night
I can see the lights of the hospital . . .
there the white hushed comings and goings,
the gray partitioning curtains,
the slow dripping in tubes.
Outside this window the last
summer flowers hemorrhage
in the gardens and winter lies
like a tumor beneath the earth.

V. Cancer and Death

In Response to a Promotional Ad Claiming that the Number of People Who Have Survived Cancer Could Now Fill the City of Los Angeles

SANDRA STEINGRABER

And the non-survivors fill the Pacific Ocean, the Grand
Canyon, and the whole of Antarctica. They fill our
silences. And they fill our mouths when we try to speak.
They inhabit vast and magnificent cities.
The non-survivors remember Los Angeles as just a dot
on the map—a stone's throw in the sticks
where everybody knew each other's business.
And then there is the wife of the man in Illinois:
he's been walking the streets for thirty years
because the space of her body fills every living room of
every house he sees.

I say whoever writes P.R. for the American Cancer Society
also writes P.R. for Dow Chemical and the Pentagon. Go talk
to the Nevada rancher who looked up at the doctor and asked,
"Who wants to survive chemotherapy just to live in L.A.?"
Let's point out that the immigration laws
in that town have not changed since 1950.
And who can sleep: the breastless, hairless ones
always scratching at the city walls, howling at the gates
all night. Everybody wants to be an angel.

The dead are smaller than us. We have to remember that.
The dead take up so little room. Their houses are modest,
they drive small cars. They've stopped dreaming
of going West.

You called this morning to say a new tumor
had flowered in your liver and another in a small coil
of the intestine. I murmured something,

promised to make a few phone calls.
I hardly know you actually. But I had mentioned once
that I was a resident of that lucky city. Sweet California.

An Interview with Claude

BRIGITTE GLUBA

Claude Delventhal's openness and her willingness to speak about her long battle with cancer were major inspirations for this volume. In May 1989, a few months before she died, she talked about how her disease affected her relationship with her children.

CD: I have two children who are twelve and fourteen years old. I was first diagnosed with cancer in 1982. That was the beginning of a long process. The children's father and I tried to include them, then six and eight, in what was going on, to explain each fear before it could overpower us. At their young ages, the children didn't have any understanding of cancer, so we told them that Mom has cancer, that she will have to go through treatments which will make her very tired, and that this is a really serious illness. The children listened, and I think they began to feel some anxiety. Each time I saw uneasiness, I tried to make them speak.

I first dealt with my cancer by undergoing traditional treatments: chemotherapy and radiation for six months. Then I went into remission for four and a half years. I think my children were able to forget a little about my cancer during that time, and so did I. But in 1987, I was diagnosed with metastasis in my hips, back and ribs, and we had to talk to the children once again. It happened that my brother-in-law was dying from AIDS then, and that period was a very unsettling one for my children, because two people to whom they were very close were facing so-called incurable illnesses at the same time.

I did some chemotherapy, but it was so disastrous that I decided to try alternative treatments. I went to Mexico, Oregon, and then southern California regularly. Each time I took those trips, my children were restless, but they knew exactly why I left and what I was going to do there. From these different places I learned what I needed to map out my own alternative treatment, which I followed for two years. I explained to my children what I was doing, particularly with the many vegetable juices. Very often, my daughter helped me make them.

I think the fear of losing their mother is definitely with them. Juliette shows her anguish by refusing to sleep at her friends' homes. She wants to be around . . . I don't know if she consciously thinks of it.

BG: She senses a danger.

CD: Yes. She's afraid of losing me. I'm not sure about my son; he uses denial a bit more. He tries not to think about it, but I know it's there for him, too. For instance, he cuts out newspaper articles about cancer for me. He does really touching things like that. The main thing I have to do with my children is to be honest. I must talk to them and let them express their feelings so they won't be blocked inside.

My friends are terrific; they are always present. I've never had to hide anything from them. I think some of them were probably afraid when I did not follow traditional treatments and went to unofficial clinics, but out of respect for me, they never mentioned it. They have given me encouragement and support, proof of love and respect. It would be very difficult without them.

BG: Do you feel lucky, or do you think that you induced this loyalty?

CD: Things probably work both ways. There is something in me which makes it easy for them to accept me, and my choices. I also have a really good support system in the cancer community. Several years ago, I began a women's cancer support group, one of the first created outside a hospital in the Bay Area. There was a great need for that group. This small group still meets in Berkeley and has given birth to the Women's Cancer Resource Center in Oakland which Jackie Winnow started in 1987. The Center now offers referral services, information on alternative therapies, and many support groups that meet particular needs.

BG: You say that for many years you've been fighting death. Can you speak of your fears, your denial and your acceptance— how you are preparing?

CD: I often think about it. My attitude varies. When I do my meditation and my spiritual practice, I think of death with serenity; the idea doesn't bother me. I can live with it. I made spiritual friends with my fear of death. When I'm in contact with my spiritual side—which means I'm centered on it—I'm really listening to a higher power. I feel the divine side in me. I meditate—I practice meditation and visualization—and I come to an acceptance which doesn't eliminate the struggle. The struggle is simply to do the footwork, to do what I have to do daily. Alternative methods take a lot of time; I mean, shopping for organic vegetables, preparing juices and special meals, taking all my medications, going to the acupuncturist, massages, meditation group, meetings, etc. All that takes practically all my time. I also want to spend time with my children. I'm constantly busy. For two years it was my full-time job to heal myself. Then, I became very bored and depressed taking care of my health. Coincidentally, I began to get worse. I left for a month in Martinique to get away from this reality. It was sunny, and there was nothing around to remind me of my cancer. I felt completely free and well after one week, and I lived my life day by day. Now that I'm back I have to be careful not to fall again into the same depression. I just had new tests which showed that I have to do some radiation, so I started yesterday. I also took steps to find a part-time job. I hope when my treatment is over I'll be able to work, and that is really frightening because after so many years I feel that I have forgotten everything, that I won't be good enough. It's both hard and important to me to participate in stimulating intellectual and social activities.

BG: So you are looking for a job, you are doing radiation therapy, and you are continuing your alternative treatments.

CD: More or less. I have to change my diet because of the radiation, and I'm happy about that because I was getting sick of eating salad, brown rice, and cereals. When I was in Martinique, I had a diet with more protein. That worked out well for me. I'm going to continue and eat more fish and organic chicken once a week. When I allow myself to vary my diet a little bit, it is both psychologically and physically good. I don't feel so deprived. Also, radiation therapy kills a large amount of bone marrow. I'll be tired and anemic, but hopefully I will compensate the loss by eating more protein.

BG: Is there harmony among all your treatments?

CD: My doctors don't know each other. I see them as my consultants. I take what I like from each, and I combine the treatments in a way that makes sense to me. The radiation will take six more weeks, and then I hope to go on vacation.

BG: Did you talk to your children about these treatments?

CD: Yes. I also brought home a video explaining what radiation is. You see, right now I have nausea due to the radiation.

BG: You said that you have many friends who support you, but you also talked about lonely moments. Would you go further?

CD: Lonely moments. Sometimes in the middle of the night, when there is no friend around. This illness threatens your life. There are frightening, anguished moments that are really difficult to share. Sometimes I tell some people, but sometimes I don't. I try to remember that the anguish will disappear, because it will, especially with spiritual help. But the idea of leaving my children is really hard. This is the hardest. I can't bear to think of my children's grief.

BG: You have your own story with your mother as a reference.

CD: Yes. My mother died at forty-eight. I'm forty-three. I don't know if I'll make it to forty-eight. My relationship with my mother was completely different from mine with my children. My mother and I were not close. I was in a boarding school all the time, and she died when I was sixteen, before we established a closeness. I didn't feel her death except in dreams, you see. Otherwise, I completely blocked it out. I began to cry for my mother's death ten years after it happened. I hope my own children can and will be encouraged to express what they have to. I really would like them to work with a counselor, someone they know and who knows them and can help them face their loss . . . you know . . . avoid the pretense that nothing has happened.

BG: This has to do with your own grief ten years after your mother's death?

CD: It has to do with what is sane and what is not. I mean, when we live something, it is sane to feel instead of not to. Feel and express what we feel, then heal. But if we don't feel, we never heal.

BG: Have you prepared your children for that time?

CD: I haven't done it because at the moment I don't feel close to death. I will do it when death gets closer, I'm sure.

BG: In any case, you have developed a different relationship with your children than the one you had with your mother.

CD: Yes, completely different. I've been so prudent. I had my children relatively late, after I'd already done some psychotherapy and examined my relationship with my mother. I was really aware that I did not want to replicate that relationship. I've avoided imposing on my children the guilt that I felt when I was a child. They have a safe environment and my unconditional love. They have the freedom to express their feelings instead of having to swallow them like I did.

BG: Do you think it works?

CD: It seems to. Sometimes I'm afraid for Juliette because she has almost lost me so many times, because she lost her uncle. There are times when she is very vulnerable. Sometimes she is afraid during the night. She's afraid to lose people, and she's working on this issue with a counselor at school. She has a tendency to want to help everybody, to be really involved in others' business. That disturbs me a bit because I recognize myself in it—helping, rescuing others.

BG: You're present, you teach her, you try to show her.

CD: I try, yes. My cancer taught me to take care of myself. I had to get cancer to learn. Before, I didn't know what it meant or how to do to it; I never felt, when I was a child, that I was worth being taken care of. I was not taught how to take care of myself, and yet, when my mother died, I had to take care of my younger brother. I became a mother then. In my relationships, I often took care of the other and abandoned myself. I didn't explore who I was, what I wanted to do. I didn't think it important.

It took cancer for all this to change, because I had to be completely dedicated to myself. It has been a strange apprenticeship, but I think that I've learned well. I've learned a bit of selfishness.

BG: It is without doubt really important. You said that your children's uncle was ill, too. He had AIDS and died two years ago. At the same time, your remission was over.

CD: He was the first person they know who died. I found a small, cancerous cyst under my arm a few days after Kent informed us that he had AIDS. His illness was really devastating for me. I loved him a lot. He had a strong attitude, no denial. He knew that he was going to die. He arranged not to be taken by force to a hospital where he might get inhumane treatments which did nothing. He didn't wish to be prolonged that way. He approached his death very rationally. He was not spiritual; he was a materialist in his approach. He thought it was a coincidence when a person falls ill. When I was diagnosed with bone cancer, he said to me, "Claude, if I could go instead of you, take your illness, I'd do it because I don't have children." He said to me that he would like to have my cancer.

He prepared for his death. He was part of a euthanasia group. I don't know if it's legal, but someone can find help to commit suicide in an easy way if she or he is going to die. Actually, I don't think he committed suicide. He had a peaceful death at home. We found him asleep on his bed next to his dog. It looked like he had died in his sleep. Nobody thought of suicide, even though he was part of the euthanasia group.

BG: Do you think of such preparation for yourself?

CD: This morning I was listening to Barbara: "Le jour de mon enterrement . . ." [The day of my burial . . .] I want that song on my burial day.

BG: I remember last time you had chemotherapy. I came to see you one day, and you were really sick. You said you wanted to stop it all. You suffered too much. It was unbearable. Impossible. You began going to Mexico for alternative treatment. You stopped the chemotherapy. What will you do if you're told that you need chemotherapy again?

CD: They already told me that a few months ago.

BG: Will you consider, as Kent did, the possibility of suicide? How do you plan for a future when you might be really sick?

CD: If it were the end, I would take strong painkillers. I would try to be as comfortable as I can for the rest of my days, but I would not like to die in a hospital. I would not want to be given chemotherapy or operated on when I'm obviously dying already. I would not want to submit myself to that. I would rather go away peacefully.

BG: We talked about many things: death, your relationships with your children, your friends. How do you like to think of your life since 1982?

CD: I have learned a lot from this disease. I learned to be in touch with myself, to love myself much more. I discovered more of who I was, who I am. I've changed; I'm not the same person who got sick. I don't feel alone right now. I know that I can always ask for help, courage, and strength. I have all the strength I need in me. It's right there.

I go through pain and try to make life as comfortable for myself as I can. I feel nourished by the love of my family and friends. I don't usually feel alone, even though it is often hard to deal with the feelings of loss, fear, sadness, anger that come up. And I have moments of peaceful happiness and pure joy.

Claude died in November 1990 at home—as she wished, with family and friends there.

Sanctuary

MARSHA CADDELL MATHEWS

Driven by cancer's dark-winged threat,
she finds her way to a forbidden shore
where thousands of seabirds
nest in the underbrush.
This time, it's the human
who's out of place—
no highways or highrises, here.
Only scrub palm and sea oats
and the calls of a thousand gulls.

Here death seems a natural thing:
cartilage, sand, and eggshell—one,
she can almost forget
the cool tubular stuff of hospitals.

On the beach
shipwrecked memories wash jagged rocks.
A white-faced pelican swoops down,
its pouch a loose-skinned rumple.
On fat webbed feet, it flip-flaps
up to her. She strokes its wing,
pallid but warm
against her open hand.

Practicing Eternity

CAROL GIVENS

*This is the story of my experience with illness and
facing death. I know my story is not unique, but as
I think about life and try to prepare for death, I find
that there are very few people willing to discuss this
process. I have some ideas about what happens when
one dies, and I have been searching for some written
trace of other women like myself. Like so many other
women's stories, the stories of lesbians facing terminal
illness are still well hidden. Lesbians live in a
subculture, and it seems we die there, too.*

August, 1987: I am going through a lot of emotional changes
right now. Lately I have experienced moments of utter numbness, as if one more thought or word about myself would put me
over the edge. My body is reacting; I am uncomfortable in it.
Uneasiness, muscle tension, leg cramps. And tired.

I don't know; maybe I really am okay after all. And maybe the
added drama of receiving a' terminal diagnosis is nothing more
than a piece of information for me to use in my life. I have always
tended to look forward to an easier time when things would be
better. So maybe I need to learn how to be alive and enjoy today,
regardless of the circumstances and without dreaming of the better
possibilities of tomorrow.

December, 1987: Time seems to go ever so slowly. Then suddenly
it is forever gone, in big chunks. The days go slowly; it's the
years that zip by. I am scared. I look in the mirror and see dark
circles under my eyes, feel how tired I am, and I wonder if I will
ever feel really well again. I wonder if I will ever have energy
to spare or feel like running in the Bay to Breakers. I keep finding
references to or obituaries of people dying "after a long illness."
Or, as I saw yesterday, a reference to someone who "finally
succumbed to cancer after a battle of two years." I'm not really
conscious of the success cases; I keep seeing where it all started

going downhill with the first diagnosis. Feeling okay for a while, but then it comes back again. Like the first thought the first time: This is the beginning of the end.

This is one of the myths about cancer—that everyone dies. Not everyone dies. There are plenty of people walking around who have been told they were terminal at some point in their lives. But I keep thinking that they have some inner will to hang in there with life that I don't have. It's not that I have nothing to live for. I mean, I don't have to get my kids through school or anything like that, but there are a lot of things that we talk about doing. There is still so much love and time to have with Diane. She reminds me about our dreams of growing old together; yet I have always been afraid of growing old, of not being able to take care of myself. Afraid of depending on others. I see other people who are sick and have been sick a lot longer than I have. How do they keep going? Susan quotes her mother, who says she just keeps on doing and can't understand why everybody is writing her off.

I do enjoy life. I appreciate nature, the talents I have, the love in my life, the people around me, the animals. How lucky I am in so many ways. I do experience joy, and still I am tired. But how to ever explain this to Diane? All she knows is that I may leave her here, and that makes her very angry. I know I would be angry were the situation reversed. Yet we are learning to be very open with one another. Getting away from the "dark" side that we are afraid to show.

February, 1988: Fran died. She was a member of the Cancer Support Group, and she had a brain tumor. She and I were the only ones who had terminal diagnoses when Diane and I started the group. So there was some kind of bond between us. She had not been to the group for a while, and I hadn't spoken with her lately. Finding out that she had died affected me greatly. I felt I had gotten much from her during the group meetings. I will miss her. I also feel like I'm next. Next in line to die. I am certainly far from death at this point, but it reaffirmed for me that, yes, people do die from cancer. Everyone else is going through treatments and getting good test results and doing great. My last CT scan showed how much worse my tumor is.

I had to go to Social Services at Community Hospital today. Walking down the hallways and looking into patients' rooms brought on this terrible fear. I do not want to go back into the hospital for anything. I hadn't felt that before. So I got kind of freaked out. I am tired of all these problems, of my bladder not working, of my colon not working, of pain, of reactions to drugs, etc., etc. I am damn sick and tired of the AMA approach to dealing with terminal illness: alleviate the pain, fix the colon, take care of each problem as it arises, but don't inspire any hope of real recovery or change.

April 9, 1988: Pain. Bone-wrenching pain. Nothing like pain to start your day out right. Each morning this week I have waked in pain, not able to lie in bed one moment longer. I practically jump up, just to stand. To do anything other than lie down on that hip of mine one more instant. Standing isn't that great, either. As I write this I am kneeling on a cushion. Sitting is not comfortable. Leave it to me to get a tumor in my butt.

April 12, 1988: Hallelujah! It appears that my bladder is going to function on its own, at least for the time being. I have been praying for some sign of healing to occur. Not that I am expecting miracles overnight, but it is so reassuring to see something hopeful. I've become so sensitive to medical people acting like they just want to make me as comfortable as possible until I die. I am not going to die! There is too much for me to do yet.

June, 1988: Woke up today feeling fear—fear of tumor growth, fear of the fear causing more tumor growth. I have had more feelings of pressure in my whole pelvic area, making it increasingly more difficult to sit; I am kneeling as I write. Pain. What can be said about pain? It is ever present to some degree. It keeps me from really experiencing the moment a lot of the time because my awareness is there, on the tumor, with the pain, rather than with what is going on in my life. When there isn't really pain, there is the pressure. The pressure of having something growing inside my abdomen. Of this mass pressing on my organs, my bowels, my bladder, and my nerves. Sending signals of a burning sensation or numbing me out completely. A large area of my right hip and thigh is numb. Feels very strange. The first thing I am aware of in the morning, and the last thing at night: pain.

November, 1988: I'm waiting for some nurses from Home Ed who will perform a procedure that consists of installing a semi-permanent line into my vein for the morphine so that I will have pain control for the rest of my days. We found out yesterday that my time may be a little more limited than we had previously thought. It appears that my tumor is impinging on my bowel at this point and is giving me a partial obstruction now, and soon may become a total obstruction. This means I can't eat any more. There are ways of keeping people alive by intravenous tubing, but that causes complications and doesn't last very long. You have to change the site every three days; you run out of sites; you run into problems with your lungs collecting fluids. My one kidney may become overtaxed. My liver is probably already overtaxed from all the morphine I've taken for so long. I'm not a good candidate for surgery, needless to say. It looks like the way to go is to just starve myself over the next few weeks. I'll just gradually get weaker and weaker and go into a coma, and soon be gone.

There is so much that I want so many people to know, and I don't know if I'll have the time, or the clarity, to let them know everything. I want Diane to know that I love her like no human being could ever love another, but I think she is aware of that. Funny; I feel a softness towards everything and everybody. I don't know if it's this sense of comfort which comes from knowing what's happening, but it's a wonderful feeling. It's too bad it only comes at this stage of the game. I sound like the voice of doom, don't I? Who knows how long I may have; but I keep learning something new every day. Learning about the world I live in and the people I live with. I'm appreciating people like never before. I'm smiling—smiling a lot. I hope that I'll be able to maintain clarity enough to finish this journal. That's the main thing for me right now. I want to feel that I have been able to complete this undertaking that Diane and I have begun together. It's exciting to think about leaving something behind that might be useful to others.

As it gets closer to the end, people are starting to say goodbye. It is such a difficult process, getting ready to say goodbye. It's a formidable task to hold up emotionally while going through this. How do you say goodbye permanently? There are things I want people to know, and people tell me things they would never ordinarily tell me, which is kind of interesting. A friend said that she and another woman who know Diane and me have always talked about our relationship and about how much we have and share. They say they have envied us.

Well, there is little more to tell, so I will end this journal now. Diane has a list of people to call when I'm gone. I do hope it doesn't take anyone totally by surprise. They have all been caring and loving, and I am so very grateful.

Carol Givens died on January 12, 1989. She was thirty-six.

Images of Dying

BARBARA ROSENBLUM

Today is January 7, 1988. Two days ago, my doctor told me that I have between three and five months to live, maybe a little less. That's about 100 to 150 days. About a quarter of a year. About 3,000 hours.

I have a very aggressive breast cancer which has already spread to my liver and to my lungs. The cancer has been successfully controlled for the past three years with surgery, radiation and chemotherapy, techniques otherwise known as slash, burn and poison. But cancer cells have a property that makes cure impossible in my case as well as in many other cases: the cells are smart little fuckers and go so far as to change their own genetic structure so that they can survive and multiply in even the most adverse environments.

I am now dying. There is no treatment for me any more. In the future, there will be other kinds of drugs called biological enhancers, drugs like interferon and interleukin, that stimulate the immune system to fight the cancer. Doctors will be able to offer newer treatments with fewer side effects. But it is not the future yet.

Today I called the hospice of San Francisco. Next week, I'll have an intake interview. They will assign a hospice worker to my case, someone who has experience with the dying. That person will help with medical and social needs. Already I have begun to see that the process of dying can benefit from the intervention and assistance of those with professional expertise.

These are the facts at this moment. Is it possible to document these fleeting facts? If you were a photographer in this room with me, you might begin to document this terminal phase of my life by showing changes in my habits and my body over time. If you want to be anthropological about it, you might decide to use "scientific" sampling. This is a method often used by social scientists who want to use visual media to study and document aspects of human life. Instead of photographing me whenever you feel like it, you set up a "shooting" schedule and take pictures at certain specified time intervals on a regular basis. Let's say, for example, that you'll take eight shots at 9 a.m., eight at 1:30 p.m. and eight at 8 p.m. That's twenty-four exposures, black and white, one roll a day.

As time passes and the disease infiltrates my body more and more, the content of the snapshots will change. Let's take, for example, the 9 a.m. pictures. At first the pictures will show a bright, spunky woman walking her dog or eating a big breakfast of ham and eggs, complete with cups of steaming coffee made from first-class beans ground only moments before filtering. Or perhaps the pictures will show me sitting at the typewriter, looking intense and full of concentration, pounding energetically, trying in a last-minute attempt to fix the words to the page.

Three weeks later, the 9 a.m. pictures will be different. Breakfast may be a small bowl of porridge, and I may be sitting at the table in my bathrobe rather than my daily clothing. There are no more pictures of me walking the pooch. I now pace around the apartment. It's safer, and when my breath runs out, I lie down until I can catch my breath once again. The hilly, slanted streets of San Francisco, the ones that look so good in chase scenes in Hollywood movies, are too hard for me now. But there's still a picture of me sitting at the typewriter.

Another three weeks pass. The 9 a.m. images are different yet again. I sit at the table in my bathrobe, staring at the glass of orange juice and the anti-nausea pill. The next image shows me struggling to get it down. Now I seldom walk around the apartment. Even that is too tiring. Staying in bed is easier, and I can breathe more easily by lying flat so that my swollen liver does not push against my diaphragm, decreasing the amount of air I can inhale. The swelling in my abdomen is now visible. I look pregnant, but I am merely filled with fluids that no longer pass into the liver but collect stagnantly in the abdominal tissues. This swelling is the first visible physical sign of my illness. All the other images in your photographs have merely shown differences in my behaviors. There are no pictures any more of me at the typewriter. Instead, I write in bed on the lap desk given to me by a friend on my last visit to England.

Four weeks later, I am sleeping at 9 a.m. If the film were color, it would show yellowed eyes and a yellow tone to my skin. Liver malfunction manifests itself as jaundice. In one picture, my left eyelid is lifted slightly, a sign that I understand that I am being photographed but that I am too weak to speak or interact or perhaps even to care. Three days later, I am dead. I am forty-five years old.

Take the pictures, put them in time sequence. What do we have? We have a 9 a.m. view of human life, an impoverished account, a too-narrow sampling of all the possible events, interactions, emotions and expressions. There's something missing. Two elements immediately come to mind. One consists of all the moments, all the possibilities, all the expressions which have been omitted, a photographer's time-honored approach towards the subject premised on "capturing the decisive moment," in Henri Cartier-Bresson's words. The second ingredient that's missing is my subjectivity.

Let's correct the first flaw by rewriting the shooting scenario, but this time changing one major assumption. Instead of doing "scientific" documentary photography, the photographer will shoot based on inspiration, mood, interaction with me, the quality of our connectedness. This time the photographer wants to capture the feelings, the expressions, and the emotions which are available, instead of just capturing a chain of events and varying habits and behaviors. This time the photographer wants to include many more possibilities. This time the photographer documents my interaction with friends and moments of solitude. This time the pictures of my face reveal the agitation, calm, panic, anxiety or shyness that I feel.

The difference between the first and second methods of documentary photography derives from the two different types of sampling techniques. The first is highly selective sampling; the second can be construed as "exhaustive" sampling. One style yields a narrow slice of reality, whereas the other yields a far richer, far more varied and complex landscape.

But missing from documentary photography, no matter how frequently or infrequently the photographer may be inspired, is my subjectivity. Can my subjectivity ever be made visible or be given a material form by a person who is not me?

One way to approach this dilemma involves interviewing the person who is photographed, recording sentences and transcribing statements, putting them into an edited form of text to accompany the photographs. Sometimes the statements are typed crudely, giving them one type of authenticity; sometimes, especially for books and gallery shows, the statements are typeset and enlarged, giving them an air of authority. The problem is—stated very simply—that once the utterances are transformed into text, they are objectified. They are no longer the stuff of subjectivity.

Perhaps it would be better to have a tape recorder running while showing the photographs. The sound of the spoken word, the tenor of my voice, my words spoken from my own emotions, my own rhythms and cadences, are so different from words on a page. I know. All of my life I have written for the page, recorded words and paragraphs for the eyes to swallow, and only now do I understand anything at all about the import of the human voice making sounds and speaking. Words-as-text without the sound of my voice have now become, for me, dead language.

Let's say we use a tape recorder and hear my voice with the accompanying photographs. Does this now solve the problem posed by subjectivity? Well, yes and no. I have told you something meaningful about myself and I have revealed something about my internal life to another person, actions which arise from my subjectivity. In the sense that words about my internal feelings and pictures of me have now been used to represent me and a time period in my life, they now enter the doubtfulness and discourse of representation. Do I really look like a dying person? Which picture is the "best" picture of a dying person? Don't we have ideal pictures in our collective cultural mind that best represent the dying? And what about the sentiments? Should some phrases on the tape make us weep and cry with sorrow? What does a person facing death talk about? Aren't some statements more appropriate to a dying person than others? What words and images are the best combination to represent a dying being?

My emotions change rapidly, they rise and fall, become transformed, go in circles and come out squares. I go from sorrow to joy to anxiety to calm all in five minutes. The rapid oscillation of my interior emotional life does not easily yield to expression and representation. Furthermore, the emotional accompaniments of the images you shoot don't lend themselves to materialization. How can you convey the awful helplessness I experience when I must take medicine because of nausea or pain? How can you know the shame and embarrassment I experience when you ask me if it's okay to photograph my swollen stomach, bursting with its enlarged liver and liquids that are dammed up and not flowing properly? How can I tell you about the shyness I've always had about my body, especially now that my figure has been altered by the effects of chemotherapy, now that my body seems misshapen? The camera by its very nature demands exposure, demands that I open to it. Subjectivity, by its nature, demands that I shut everything and everyone out so that I can hear myself. I find myself placed squarely in a contradiction between the objectifying nature of representation and the requirements of quiet and solitude in order to successfully stay alive to the subjectivity in myself.

I think subjectivity matters because it attempts to give meaning to the actions and behaviors of the actors. Without knowing how they individually experience the world, how they see and interpret things, we viewers are forced to rely on only our own interpretations of their behavior. Subjectivity particularizes.

The camera, however, is a universalizing instrument despite the uniqueness and specificity of each image and each person. It uses the particular to make the general message effective. In a specific face, we think we see "people." Photography feeds back information about what it means to be a human being, not just in this moment or in this time or among this class of people. It sweeps us up into its humanizing grasp, leaving the viewer with a tentative and ambiguous understanding of the relations between the specific and the universal.

I have a few more things to say. The images you take of me look too banal, too trivial, too individualized to mean anything significant. You don't show my entire history, and even if you did, it still would remain stuck on the individual level. You can't show the history of breast cancer because, first, it's impossible. Secondly, such an endeavor would be a historical project, not the portrayal of an individual life. Yet, without the historical frame of reference, my individual story suffers from lack of fuller meaning. Without my individual story, a historical pictorial essay on breast cancer suffers from lack of specificity, the absence of a single person with whom the viewer can identify and thereby experience emotion. An unhistoricized version of my life, whether my individual life or the history of the illness I have, is vulnerable to a representation that may rely on culturally common stereotypes in order to make its points. Lacking specificity but seeking universality, an image can devolve into a cultural cliché.

Let's say everything I've written so far are the angry, crusty protests of someone who won't have much more time to make pictures and write words. Let's say you're a photographer and I'm your assignment. There's only one way to find out. Give me a call.

Why Don't You Just Die?

DEBORAH SMITH

Aren't you dead yet?
I bought you flowers
    I sent you a card
        I said my condolences
We had a wonderful, healing communication
Truth is, *you* inspired *me*
I was amazed by your calm, optimistic demeanor
How cool you were in the face of this tragedy
For a moment I glimpsed something big
    I saw and felt the transience of life

Then I went back to my life
The day-to-day trivialities captured me
    and held me hostage

I heard you were still alive
    Not recovered, no remission, but still hanging on

I have nothing to say to you now
I gave you what I could
Why don't you just die so I can go on with my life
and be free of your haunting memory?

VI. Living in Cancer's Shadow

Not Yet Cancer

HOLLY O.

A lot of people get cancer these days. One-third of Americans will eventually get cancer. Every year nearly a million people will be diagnosed with cancer and nearly half of those people will lose their lives to it within five years. Every year half a million people will die from cancer.[1] The remaining millions, the millions who don't yet have cancer, comfort themselves by being certain that cancer won't happen to them; cancer only happens to other people. But some of those millions of people who don't yet have cancer can't rest so easily—some of us live very intimately with a threat of cancer which is much more real than any statistical probability.

Cancer sits right next to me every hour of every day. Five years ago I was diagnosed with cervical dysplasia, a pre-cancerous condition. Dysplasia, an "abnormal development of tissue,"[2] is one of those ailments that you discover only through a test result. There are no telltale symptoms: no headache, no pain, no lump, no rash. Cervical dysplasia simply means "bad cervical cells," a condition uncovered by a Pap smear.

Sometimes, however, there are bothersome vaginal infections which might indicate that dysplasia is alive and well. I am always waiting for these infections, always anxious, always focused in some way or another on my pelvis. Just recently I discovered a yeast infection on the Saturday morning of a long weekend. By that evening I could hardly stand the itch, but I knew no doctor would see me until Tuesday. I scanned through the women's medical books and herbal remedy guides I've collected since discovering my illness. Several suggested acidophilus-yogurt douches as a home remedy for yeast infections.

I drove all over town that Saturday night in a frenzy, looking for yogurt and acidophilus capsules to mix with it. After tromping through at least half a dozen open-all-night grocery stores, I found the acidophilus capsules. I took them home, along with a carton of yogurt, and mixed the concoction in my kitchen at 1:00 in the morning. I spent a glorious three-day weekend lying down on my bathroom floor at four-hour intervals trying to spoon acidophilus-spiked yogurt into my vagina.

Every time I notice the slightest difference in how I feel—an itch or a pain or a discharge—I panic. Is this a simple yeast infection, or is it this time something more serious? And even if it is only a yeast infection, is it a yeast infection of and unto itself, or is it a warning signal that the dysplasia is kicking in again? And when there is dysplasia, is it only a result of the yeast infection, or is the dysplasia causing the yeast infection? And will the dysplasia go away by itself, or will I have to take medicine again? Will I need surgery this time? Or is this the time—of all the times—that it is cancer?

In and of itself, dysplasia means only a few irritating infections, a few extra trips to the gynecologist each year. But dysplasia is also a precancerous condition. A class "0" or class "1" smear is normal; a class "2," "3," or "3-A" smear indicates varying degrees of dysplasia. And a class "4" smear means cancer. Depending upon which expert one talks to, the numbers between class "1" and class "4" could indicate merely infection, an abnormal cell growth, or a pre-cancerous condition. It's the pre-cancerous condition which plagues me.

The thought of cancer is terrifying. It means death, or at least serious illness, hysterectomy, radiation, chemotherapy. Yet sometimes I almost hope that my next Pap test will show that my "3-A" has turned into a "4," that my dysplasia will finally come out and show its real potential. Every year 15,000 women are diagnosed with cervical cancer,[3] and sometimes I hope that I have joined them at last, for then I could deal with it, or fight it, or have someone cut the cancer out of me. And then too, if my cervix were pronounced cancerous, my fears would finally be considered valid. I could cry and worry all I wanted or needed, and I would be perfectly within my rights.

But a threat of cancer is not "real" cancer. It is not something I can join a support group over, and even my gynecologist treats it with only mild concern. Nevertheless, cervical dysplasia for me has been a personal threat to my happiness and well-being. It has threatened my independence, my self-esteem, and my fertility.

I discovered that I had cervical dysplasia during the winter break of my freshman year of college. After my first five months away from home I was feeling proud and independent. One act of my new independence included visiting a family planning clinic in my hometown during the break to get birth control. What I got instead was a strict order to see my regular physician immediately, as my Pap smear had been rated a class "3-A."

I went to my parents in tears. I tried to explain to them what was wrong. With painful embarrassment I also had to tell my parents under what circumstances I had discovered my problem.

I thought I was dying.

My parents arranged a doctor's appointment for me right away. I got in to see one of "the best" gynecologists in the city's medical clinic. As I lay on the examining table, naked except for a paper gown, this "best" doctor brought a young male intern with him into the examination room. He hadn't asked either my permission or my parents', and the unwelcome presence of the young man certainly added to my feelings of powerlessness, fear, and invasion. After his examination, the doctor gave me a vague description of what was wrong, but I still thought I might be dying. When I expressed my worries, he told me not to concern myself. He slapped my naked thigh and said he'd have me "back to all [my] boyfriends at college in no time."

The nonchalance of doctors, hard as that is to combat, is not nearly so bad as the reactions of many people when they learn of my dysplasia. Though my family and my friends have been extremely supportive, other people have openly condemned me because of the sexually related aspects of this disease. I've been told many times, in no uncertain terms, that sexual promiscuity is the cause of cervical dysplasia and cervical cancer, even though there is no real evidence to support that claim. There is also some indication that sexual promiscuity is linked to prostate cancer, too, but a man with prostate cancer doesn't face the moral outrage and social disgrace because of *his* cancer that I face because of my dysplasia.

I remember one particular pro-choice demonstration I attended. To fuel our anger and boost our determination before our march, a speaker read to the crowd a series of quotes by well-known anti-abortionists. I laughed and shouted and clapped with the crowd at each of the outrageous statements. But then the speaker read a quote from a very well-known woman anti-abortionist which suggested that the possibility of contracting cervical dysplasia should be used as a scare tactic to warn women away from having premarital sex, because women who did have sex before marriage and had cervical dysplasia had gotten what they deserved. My spirits sank.

And while I wrestle, really wrestle, to build self-esteem and create a good feeling about my own sexuality, I hate the people who have said those things. Because even if it were true that cervical dysplasia could be linked to sexually promiscuous behavior, what difference would it make? When I found out that I had dysplasia of the cervix, I was eighteen years old and scared out of my mind. I didn't care how it started; I just wanted it over. Five years later I still struggle to get well, stay well, and battle this nonexistent cancer that is nonetheless a real threat to me. What have the judgments of these people done for me? They haven't helped me. They haven't enlightened me. They haven't given me courage or strength. Those self-righteous insinuations against my moral character have only made me feel ashamed, and they have forced me to keep my fears bottled up and sealed with silence.

I am angry at those faraway authors, doctors, and spokespeople who have hurt me so deeply and irreparably. I am angry at the medical specialists who have treated me callously and who did not acknowledge my fear. I am angrier still at the doctors who failed even to notice that I was a person.

We all live with the worry about cancer in the backs of our minds, but I might be lucky enough to never have to deal with dysplasia again. Today I am physically better than I was five years ago. This particular agony might be over for me.

And it might not.

NOTES

1. Holleb, Arthur I, ed., *The American Cancer Society Cancer Book*, Doubleday & Co., Inc., New York, 1986, pp. xvii-xviii.
2. *Taber's Cyclopedic Medical Dictionary*, 10th Edition, R.A. David Co., Philadelphia, 1965.
3. *Rachel's Hazardous Waste News*, No. 130, Environmental Research Foundation, Princeton, New Jersey, 1989.

Decisions

NICOLA MORRIS

In my dreams the beds are in rows, and I have no choice about whom I sleep next to. Everyone in the room last night had cancer, and I had a boyfriend. The room was a ward for breast cancer, and it was visiting time. The woman to the right of me was lying on her bed. Her husband came to visit, lay on top of her with all his clothes on and rested his head on her left breast. She pushed him away, and I saw that it was not her left breast, but the space where her left breast used to be. I think that possibly, though, it is not all empty space; perhaps she has some of her breast left. Perhaps just a piece of her breast was cut out.

If I get breast cancer, it will be my right breast. I inspect that breast intermittently for lumps. There always are lumps, and every year or so I panic and get a mammogram to see if there are lumps to worry about. Mammograms cause cancer too, so whether to get the X-ray is often a hard decision to make, and I get very distracted. I can't think about my job or about what to cook for dinner, because I worry about it. Shall I take this percentage of risk of getting cancer to find out if I have cancer, because if I have it and don't know about it, then there is this other percentage of risk that I might die?

In my dream, the woman to my right sleeps under a window, but because of the operation on her breast she cannot manage to open and close the window. I guess she thinks of other decisions to make. She is very angry at her husband. Her husband is confused about why she is angry, and so am I. He has come to see her, after all. I decide she is angry because she has discovered there might be more possibilities for her life than just her husband. She has spent the last few weeks watching the boyfriend of the woman on my left, and even, perhaps, watching my boyfriend. The boyfriend of the woman on my left is very handsome. He is tall and sensitive looking. He is broad shouldered and looks as if he could protect someone. Probably, however, beneath his sensitive image he is not concerned with anyone but himself.

The husband of the woman to my right has come up from New Jersey to visit her. He has a very thin face with traces of pimples which he has tried to wash away with many splashes of a strong-smelling cologne. His hair is scarce and short, and because he keeps his head on her body even when it is not on her chest, it is impossible for me to tell the color of his eyes.

This place is my home, even though I do not have breast cancer. In the hallway my boyfriend says he wants to stay the night. I don't want him to. I want my home to be my own. I want to lie under the window and feel the soft breeze on my face, and I want to think about the woman to my right, about whether she did have that breast removed, and about why she is angry with her husband. I want to lie as flat against the mattress as I can, and then to smooth the covers down over my body so there is almost no bulge to be seen.

I think now that the woman next to me really doesn't understand why she is so angry with her husband, even though she thinks about my boyfriend too. My boyfriend is a jazz musician, and he has no money right now. She hasn't seen what he really looks like, though, because I haven't yet invited him into the room. I might invite him tonight. She thinks he is a rambler, a man who goes from town to town, who plays everywhere she has wanted to travel, and who always falls into a safe bed at night.

In this dream I don't have breast cancer, but I wake up worrying about it. Why am I dreaming of cancer so often? It seems that every night I dream of someone—usually my mother—dying of cancer. In this dream the last thing I do before I leave is look around the room, look at the women in the beds all around me, and think about how they still appear so healthy. The angry woman has color in her cheeks. At least one of the women in this room is likely to die of this breast cancer that is now so new to her.

Awake in my own bed, I put my right arm over my head and rub my fingers into my right breast. I am careful not to wake my lover because I don't want to be embarrassed. The usual lumpy area on the right—the place that slips down into being my right armpit—is still lumpy, and I can feel no other lumps anywhere. I press curiously around my nipple. I can't imagine finding a lump in that pale brown area where the skin is softer than anywhere else on my body. Although I don't find any new lumps, I always worry about the lumps I have on the right side of my breast. Perhaps I should go and see the specialist. He told me I had a 50 percent chance of developing breast cancer, and he suggested that I might like to have my breasts removed so that there is no place for the cancer to grow. I decide to touch my breasts again the next time I take a bath. I will lather them first with soap so that my hands can move easily across my skin. Then maybe I will decide about the breast doctor. It is hard for me to make decisions.

Mostly They Have None

ELIZABETH BRUNAZZI

"One," I replied, and then it occurred to me that most people didn't seem to have any more than that now. "One child or none," I suggested. Her aged, paper-white face was framed by girlish, permed blond hair as unmoving as a wig. Peering up at me over the blue plastic glasses, she caught me for a second in her clear, almost colorless eyes as her lips, painted on above the shrinking natural line in dark red lipstick, came together in a little bow. "Mostly . . . ," I said, and then her lips settled like some model of a geological cataclysm, ". . . they have none."

Then she raised my left arm straight up in the air, as if coaxing it up there to salute the machinery, pressed my left breast between two cold metal plates like a quarter-pound hamburger patty, told me that I should stop breathing when she told me to, and left the room. I kept seeing my small, entrapped breast in the shape of something like a duck's bill. "Don't breathe."

When she came back to repeat the operation on the right side, I reported that this was my first mammogram, sort of like confiding to someone that you've just had your first period or wet dream. And that I had come to the institute only because my doctor had told me almost four years ago that since I was forty he thought it would be a good idea, and how everybody had them now when they reached forty, if they hadn't had one before. "All routine," he said. This information did not impress her very much. I had expected some sympathetic reply like, "Good move," or something like that. Nothing. She just raised my right arm in the air, smushed my right breast between the plates, told me not to breathe when she signaled, and left the room again. I wondered what Diana of Ephesus would have felt like getting a mammogram. The statue in the Vatican . . . her robe layered with all those animals. All those breasts. All those plates. Have to modify the machinery. How many? I never counted them. Didn't have time. Some X-ray. "Mostly they have none." Diana—"Don't breathe"—would not like that.

I did not tell her that I had finally come in after almost four years since my fortieth birthday because I kept hearing about people, women, actually, losing one here and one there, sometimes both. First it was my daughter's stepmother, then my older—just three years older—sister's best friend, and then a friend, maybe not a very close one, of my younger sister, all in a period of about three months. "An epidemic," the stepmother had said in a shaken voice when I called up to talk to my one and only daughter. "An epidemic," my daughter had echoed as soon as she got on the phone. It seemed to be getting closer and closer, faint at first, a distant thud, and now a galloping apocalypse of mutilated breasts, chests, and upper arms. Standing there in that windowless room in that ridiculous position, I felt grateful for a minute that I still had those two little, funnel-shaped wads of flesh to sandwich into the gray, glistening machine. Like the ones dangling from the belly of the she-wolf for Romulus and Remus to suck on. From my great-grandmother. Roman breasts.

My fourteen-year-old daughter's breasts are round, but she complains that they are too far apart, almost under her armpits, she said. She wanted to know if she taped them together every night, would they grow closer together so that she could have cleavage? I said I didn't think so, but she could try it. My mother, when she was nearing fifty, used to plant a triangle of Band-Aid material between her eyes at night—the triangles came in packages labelled FROWNEES—to erase the crease she had gotten there from too much frowning. In the morning the crease would have miraculously disappeared, and there would be just a flat space, but by afternoon she would have frowned too much again, and the crease, like a five-o'clock shadow, sure as sin, would be back. FROWNEES remind me of mortality. Mother Mortality. I think that I am getting one of those creases, too. I have begun to frown too much, but I haven't seen any FROWNEES around for years. Suppose I could roll my own out of any Johnson & Johnson's package. Sell them on the street. Need a vendor's license. Black market FROWNEES. If they can sell Rolex watches on 57th Street, I can sell FROWNEES.

The small white coat with the doll-baby hair reappeared through the doorway, saying that I could start breathing again—I already was—and came over to release my right breast from the equipment. Even with it out, I had the sensation that it was still caught in the machine, or in the picture, and that I would not be able to get it back for some time. Maybe they would send it back to me in the mail along with my bill or ship it off to my doctor, who would call me in to discuss the X-ray, pull my breast from a plastic container, the kind used for packaging takeout food and destroying the ozone layer, point out certain abnormalities, and then hand it back to me at the end of the consultation. I could stick it back on or put it in my bag for future use. Convenient, purse-size breasts.

Had she been thinking about me all the time she was in that dark, windowless room with the colored lights and buttons where she sees you stop breathing for fifteen seconds or so? The same colorless stare floated up near my face again and said that I should not worry about being past forty, that it was all just beginning (she did not say what), and that for herself, she felt very young. She must have been around sixty, but it was hard to tell. I thought she smiled just slightly, but maybe she didn't. "You can take a seat now with the other ladies" were her last words as she opened the door and disappeared into another room without a backward look. Exit the priestess of the mammography room.

I sat down on one of the coral plastic chairs between two other women, all three of us dressed in identical pink, paper-towel gowns. One of them, a stylish woman with a silver bob haircut, silver hoop earrings, and a tan, appeared to be flat-chested and perhaps no longer had any breasts at all. The other one, a full-figured matron in her forties with short blond hair and a perpetual smile, had breasts so large that they were falling out of the slit up the front of her paper towel. All told, there were fifteen women in the room, seated in two rows arranged back to back down the center, as if we were about to play musical chairs. Would have been a lot more fun than sitting there on those plastic chairs, shivering in the paper towels, fidgeting with watches, bracelets, earrings, and pantyhose. Just a couple of rounds. Warm us up. Aerobic musical chairs. Let's go, ladies, one-two-three-four, marching around to Mick Jagger bawling, "You start me up," which always sounded to me as if he were singing, "In-som-ni-a." I used to sing along "In-som-ni-a" for years. Think I'll request musical chairs from the people in charge of such things if I have to go back to the institute any time soon. Maybe not, though. Might make me feel terrible if I were It. The one who missed the chair.

"Alice . . . you can go now." I didn't know whether this meant I had succeeded or failed. The large blond woman with the snug paper towel and the smile told me sweetly it just meant that they didn't have to do the X-ray again. I jumped up and ran out in case someone changed her mind, jerked on my yellow T-shirt in a stall like the ones you use at a public beach, and headed for the nearest bathroom and a cigarette.

Two women wearing nearly identical outfits, black and white tweed skirts and one red and one dark coral blouse and plenty of gold jewelry, were standing in the bathroom. One was talking about what a wonderful service the institute provided, and, yes, she was living proof of this, diagnosed fourteen years ago when she had her first mammogram, and how she had lost her left breast, but, yes, it had been caught in time, and here she was, almost good as new, here she was, and no other problems, knock on wood. She came in every three months, and she and her friend met for lunch and some shopping on those days, like the day you go in for a dye job or a pedicure.

I sat on the sill of the big window, the kind with little stars running all over it so that no one can see in the bathroom, gradually enveloped in smoke about the color of the air outside. It didn't seem to bother them that I was in there for a cigarette. They looked over and smiled, as if we had all been talking to each other for a long while and had some secret or other. Caught in time? Had we all been caught in time?

I left the office building. The women I passed had no breasts, just prosthetic devices, I think they are called, beneath their executive suits and dresses, and the men, molded plastic breastplates with hair implants beneath the Brooks Brothers. All caught in time, they were still moving briskly in the direction of their offices, back from business lunches and a quick visit to a medical institute. And the arms and legs. Ears and noses. Prosthetic devices. Breasts. The statue in the Vatican I saw last year, Diana of Ephesus . . . ancient goddess with her dozens of breasts and the fish and cows and horses and birds all flowing down the cold tiers of her robe. All the women . . . dressed in red and yellow and black and white. Be with us now.

VII. Finding Our Power

On Cancer and Conjuring

JANIS COOMBS EPPS

Words are to be taken seriously. I try to take seriously
acts of language. Words set things in motion.
I've seen them doing it. Words set up atmospheres,
electrical fields, charges. I've felt them doing it.
Words conjure.[1]

Cancer is a conjuring word. Perhaps that is why my doctor did not use the word cancer when explaining my condition. Instead she told me, "Your results indicate a gross malignancy on the lower portion of your colon." I couldn't believe what she was saying.

Is she telling me that I have cancer?

"Your tests indicate that the tumor is several centimeters and is located in the lower segment of the bowel," she continued, drawing a pencil sketch of the colon which to me looked like a curvy snake poised to strike.

Is she telling me that I have cancer?

I was sure only when she began asking questions about how often I had seen blood in my stool, and whether it was bright red or dark red. I was a thirty-three-year-old black woman in my prime. I was sassy, and thought I was fine! I was a dissertation away from a doctoral degree and was a college professor. I applauded myself for owning my own home, and single-handedly raising two bright, beautiful children after a tumultuous divorce; I also had a steady boyfriend who treated me like royalty.

Now, some black woman doctor no older than I was saying something about an operation that might save my life, and tumors and malignancies and carcinomas.

All I heard was the conjuring word: cancer. Pictures of things dark and evil-spirited possessed me. Images of withered, skeletal fingers. Empty eyes in deep, hollow sockets. Decay. Death. Cancer. I couldn't get the word out of my head. Over and over again I repeated the word silently. And every time I heard it, it was as if two great, clashing cymbals collided next to my eardrums; every vibration was a reiteration of cancer, cancer, cancer, until the sound was small and weak and barely audible. But then the clash would come again, crashing thunderously throughout my being; the word and its reality engulfed me. I sat motionless in the middle of my hospital bed with tears streaming down my cheeks. God had played a dirty trick on me. I had cancer and I was going to die.

As my doctor talked on, matter-of-factly, about my "disease" and the possibility that I might well have to undergo a colostomy, I became silently hysterical. The tears would not stop. The room was spinning. Every now and then I would catch a phrase—artificial anus, an incision from the colon through the wall of the abdomen. Inside I was screaming, trying to drown out her words. Perhaps if I did not hear them their reality would go away. Surely God was paying me back for some terrible sin I had committed. I couldn't think of what it could be, but He knew how vain I was, how important it was for me to be considered pretty. And now this doctor was talking about my wearing a hideous bag for the rest of my life—a disgusting thing to be worn on the outside of my body to hold my bodily waste.

This lady can't be for real.

For the next few days I was in shock. Not the stupefied shock of silence, but the shock of mindless chatter that hides what is really in one's mind. For some reason it was important to me that I appear normal and in control. When a visitor would ask, "How are you doing?" I could hear my voice, well modulated and in control, say, "Just fine. The doctor says that the tumor is malignant, but once it is removed I should be fine."

That is what my voice said. But the ticker tape inside my head was saying, "I've got cancer and I'm going to die, so get out of my face asking me how I'm doing!"

I was angry with the world and more than anything I wanted to be alone in my misery.

As I look back to that time, I am sure that I needed to be alone. Fundamentally I am a loner anyway, although I am also a mother, daughter, sister, friend and a teacher. I spend my free time engrossed between the covers of a book, or scribbling away madly in a notebook, or viewing a movie in a darkened theater. So the way I live my life is the way I chose to handle its tragedy—alone. Audre Lorde has said that "each woman responds to the crisis that cancer brings to her life out of a whole pattern, which is the design of who she is and how her life has been lived. The weave of her everyday existence is the training ground for how she handles crises."[2]

Whenever I am in a crisis state I have a need to curl up in the fetal position and think or not think. It is the way I heal myself. Being in a hospital was at odds with my own healing methodology, for hospitals don't allow for aloneness. Someone is always coming in to take temperatures, test urine, take blood and give shots. Doctors make rounds, friends visit, families hold hands and love you. I needed time to myself to comfort me.

But how do you tell those who love you, who are going through their own pain at the thought of losing you, that at such a critical time you don't want their physical presence? You don't tell them. Instead you act pleased that they are there offering their support. You chat courteously with the hospital staff. You welcome friends—always smiling and talking, but never mentioning the word: cancer.

Secretly I wished that they would all go away. That I could throw the flowers and the dish gardens through the hospital windows. That I could strut down that hospital hall with my hands on my hips and indiscriminately curse anybody who happened to get in my way. I needed to be loud and boisterous like a woman possessed. I didn't need anybody's pity, and I needed to show myself that I was in charge of my own life. I wanted to point my finger and shake my head and shout that cancer didn't rule me. I was mad!

But cancer is a conjuring word with powers of its own, and it didn't care whether I was mad or not. It was out to get me. Either I had an operation, or I died.

I am told that the doctors wrestled seven hours in the operating room seizing and removing the power that cancer had over my colon. Still they were not sure. So radiation and chemotherapy were scheduled. "Not immediately," I heard them say. "When she has been released from the hospital and is stronger."

My memories of the six weeks I was hospitalized following the surgery are vague, perhaps due to the drugs I was taking, or maybe because I have chosen to forget. I can remember vaguely the sensation of hips numbed by numerous injections. I'd ring the bell for the nurse. "Is it time for my shot yet?" I'd ask anxiously. "Not yet. In a little while. Just hold on," the white-clad figure would say.

Please bring my shot. I can deal with the pain from the surgery, but I need the shot to anesthetize my brain, so I don't have to think anymore.

Yet that is all I did: think. I cannot count the number of times I feigned sleep so I would not have to talk with anyone. Excuses were made for my rudeness when I ignored family and friends. A psychiatrist was called in because my depression was so severe. He was a kind, sensitive man who told me in a quiet way that I must eventually accept and deal with the fact that I had cancer. I said, "I know you are right. I must plan for my life and for my death." But inside I thought: "You must be out of your mind if you think I'm going to accept this! You say I have cancer. I say I *had* cancer."

I think the real story of the healing process from my bout with cancer starts here—whether to allow the conjuring powers of the word *CANCER* to possess and define me. I could either live my life as a cancer victim, making all my decisions based on that reality, or I would press on with my life as I was accustomed to living it. If I could control nothing else in my world, I would at least control the way I thought.

From the moment I truly realized that I might die, or might possibly spend the rest of my days with a bag hooked to my side, I had felt totally out of control, as if some force outside of me was determining my destiny. That is always the way it is. We are never totally in charge. But when we are healthy, we rarely consider the role of fate in our lives. We make our own decisions and take charge of our lives, so we think. After my operation it was clear that "the others" had wrested control of my reality. I ate and got out of bed on their schedule, had to be helped to the bathroom, and I was told that I was not to walk the halls alone because I was too weak. Outwardly, I appeared to be a good patient, doing exactly what they asked, but all the time I was going deeper into myself. For the six weeks I was hospitalized I did not look at a complete television program; I did not read a book; I did not thumb through a magazine. I simply lay there. It was my way of rebelling. "They" might control my physical reality, but "they" could not control the *me* that dwelled deep within.

I could talk to everybody on one level and think my own thoughts on another level. I had stumbled upon a way to deal with the horrors that were happening to my body. I saw myself as being separate from my body. "Janis, we can't determine why your temperature is so high. Another operation may be necessary."

Fine. I'm not really here. This is just my body.

"Janis, you're losing so much weight we may have to put a hole in your shoulder and feed you through a tube."

Hey, knock yourself out. This ain't really me.

"Janis, just to make sure that we got it all you will have to take chemotherapy treatments over a six-month period."

So what? This is just my flesh.

Most of the time I was scared, but I could deal with the fear by not defining myself as this cancerous bedridden specimen. The real me was unaffected.

Once I had worked out the distinction between my body and the real me, my greatest fear became the thought of losing my children. More than anything else in my life, I love my children. So I made numerous bargains with God that if I was allowed to live to see them reach adulthood, I would become the "perfect" person. My greatest fear was that my bargain would not be honored, and my children would not have me. I was sure that they would be loved and taken care of, but they wouldn't have me. They would not be privy to my thoughts, my ideas, my guidance. I knew that nobody could raise them like I could.

As my three-year-old daughter sat on my lap one Sunday during visiting hours, I became so choked up I could not speak. I could not leave her. She was too little to be motherless. My ten-year-old son was in the joke-telling phase of childhood, and seemed oblivious to my gloomy mood. He was simply happy that he and I could hug each other and spend some time together. He continued to tell one joke after another and to laugh hysterically after each. As I half listened to "Why did the chicken cross the road? To get to the other side. Yuk, yuk!" I knew that he would make it—even without me. He had my strength and sensitivity, and I felt he had been exposed to me long enough for me to be a part of every facet of his character. I did not feel that I had yet imprinted myself on my daughter in the same way. I couldn't let go. I had so much more love to give.

There is not much more to tell. I did not have to have the feared colostomy. There was another operation, radiation and chemotherapy. But those were things which happened to my body, not to me.

It has been several years since my trauma—strong, healthy years. Years that I have watched my toddler turn into a little girl, a little girl who acts a lot like me. Years that have seen my little boy grow into adolescence and become more his own person. I am more serene and at peace with myself, having faced the reality of my own mortality, and I am anxious to get on with life.

Cancer is indeed a conjuring word. But I am no longer afraid to say the word: Cancer. Its power comes from our fear. I have faced death, and I know that when my time comes, whether I am stalked slowly by cancer or hit swiftly by a truck, I am triumphant.

NOTES

1. Bambara, Toni Cade, "What It Is I Think I'm Doing Anyhow," *The Writer on Her Work*, Janet Sternberger, ed. W. W. Norton & Co., New York, 1980, p. 163.
2. Lorde, Audre, *The Cancer Journals*, Aunt Lute Books, San Francisco, 1980, p. 9.

Lesbians Evolving Health Care: Cancer and AIDS

JACKIE WINNOW

One of our local newspapers recently ran an article addressing the plight of the 100 women with AIDS in the San Francisco Bay Area.[1] According to the article, the local community had responded by starting many different sorts of services for these women: housing, child care, a day-care center, haircuts, a food bank, massage, counseling, meals, and other support services.

At the same time (1988), there were approximately 40,000 women living in the Bay Area with cancer. At least 4,000 of them were lesbians. In that same year, 8,000 women were newly diagnosed with cancer, and 4,000 women in the San Francisco Bay Area died from cancer.[2]

The 40,000 women with cancer don't have the services available to the 100 women with AIDS. Certainly the women with AIDS should have their services, but the very existence of those services brings into sharp focus another problem.

I am both a cancer activist and an AIDS activist. As a lesbian feminist, I have been involved with the AIDS crisis since the early 1980s. In 1985 I was diagnosed with breast cancer, founded the Women's Cancer Resource Center in Berkeley, California in 1986, and was diagnosed with metastatic breast cancer in my lungs and bones in 1988. I have lost friends, acquaintances, and colleagues to cancer and to AIDS. Both of these diseases are life-threatening, and yet I have seen my community rally around one and overlook the other.

As a feminist, I know the importance of putting discussion in a historical perspective. Without that perspective, we cannot remember our intent or hold on to our vision. Without it, we cannot remember where we've been or where we're going. Without it, we lose our own political perspective and become pawns on other people's agendas.

Throughout history, the issue of women's health has been closely related to the standing of women as healers, or caregivers, as we are now called. It is interesting to note that the term "caregivers" seems to have replaced "healers," a substitution which echoes the current status of women and reflects how we think of ourselves today.

Women have not always taken a subsidiary role in society's caring for its sick. During the Middle Ages, the great lay healers, midwives, and herbalists of the day were women, and nine million witches—mostly women—were burned for healing people. As is pointed out in *Nurses, Midwives and Witches*, "It was witches who developed an extensive understanding of bones and muscles, herbs and drugs, while physicians were still deriving their prognoses from astrology and alchemists were trying to turn lead into gold."[3]

Women were the backbone of a popular health movement in the early 1800s. They believed in hygiene, bathing, loose clothes, good nutrition, and birth control. They set up their own medical schools and became doctors. Then in 1847 the American Medical Association was born, and women were expunged from the healing professions, save for midwifery, which was allowed to proliferate in Europe. All medical schools soon followed a rigid curriculum and training, and by the late nineteenth century those schools had nearly succeeded in creating a male-only medical profession, mostly made up of men from the ruling class in the service of the ruling class.

In the health care professions of today, women have been largely relegated to nursing, a role subservient to doctors. Earlier nurses had been socially regarded as prostitutes, but by the middle of the nineteenth century middle class women, like Florence Nightingale, changed the image of the nurse to one which embodied the very essence of the cultural ideal of womanhood—selfless and dedicated. Feminists of the time supported the role of women as nurturers, probably because caregiving offered women an avenue for employment. With the development of nursing as a profession for women, curing and caring became distinctly different arenas, with men as doctors curing and women as nurses caring. Once nursing was established as a responsible occupation, other acceptable professions for women developed, all stemming from her "natural" domestic role: social worker, teacher, counselor.

History does not stand still, however, and the civil rights movement of American blacks in the 1950s and 1960s brought forward once again the notions of equality, justice, liberation and self-determination. Following the civil rights movement, the women's liberation movement in the late 1960s and early 1970s roused women to renew their demands for control over their own bodies as well as over their own destinies. Instead of relying on (predominantly male) doctors for all their information, women began to discover their own bodies and determine for themselves what was best for them. Self-help classes, women-run health clinics, pamphlets and books such as the ground-breaking *Our Bodies, Ourselves*[4] appeared and proliferated. Women began entering the medical profession in larger numbers. The United States was, and probably still is, the industrialized country with the lowest percentage of women physicians.[5] Of course, the United States and South Africa are also the only industrialized countries currently without nationalized health insurance.

The demand for legal abortions began in earnest with the women's liberation movement. In 1973, the United States Supreme Court, in Roe vs. Wade, determined that abortion fell under the fourteenth Amendment to the Constitution, which embodied the concept of the right of privacy as personal liberty. With legalization, poor women got federal Medicaid funding; women health workers improved abortion techniques and set up referral services and women-controlled clinics. But, as we know, that struggle has been long and hard, and it is far from over yet.

At the same time, the lesbian and gay liberation movements also took their first steps. From the founding of the Daughters of Bilitis in the 1950s to the Stonewall Rebellion of 1969, lesbians and gay men began gaining visibility as they demanded the right to love and happiness. The recognition of the oppressiveness of a heterosexist society and the interconnections between sexism and homophobia made it clear, at least for radical lesbians, that one can't be "free" on the one hand, if not also on the other.

Lesbians have been in the vanguard of the current women's and lesbian/gay liberation movements and have held uncomfortable places in both. In the women's liberation movement, lesbians have been suspect for being lesbian, and in the gay/lesbian movement, suspect for being women. Our needs, if noticed at all, are placed on the back burners of the agenda makers. We were always the other in the lesbian/gay and women's movements, although we were often the exciting and driving energy in both.

I began to work on the AIDS crisis in 1982 when AIDS hysteria endangered our civil rights, increased anti-lesbian/gay violence, divided our community over the bathhouse and sexuality issues, and increased discrimination, particularly in the area of employment. AIDS hysteria and misinformation caused great numbers of men—in a community of people already considered to be pariahs—to question their gayness, their sexuality and their self-esteem. While little was firmly known about the cause or transmission of AIDS, it was clear that large numbers of gay men were getting it, and that our survival as a people depended on our response. And we, the lesbian/gay community, reacted admirably—with vigor, courage and caring.

As a community, we had never before received much funding for any of our organizations or services. Much of our early organizing was grassroots, and we had little concrete experience for what was to come, though our past work laid a solid foundation upon which to respond to this crisis. From next to nothing, we created services that educated the lesbian/gay and general communities, housed people with AIDS/ARC, served them meals, provided emotional and practical support, and provided funds. We created model programs for hospital care, hospice care, and social services. We demanded government responsiveness, fought for good legislation, and continue to fight tirelessly against bad legislation and bigotry. We created information services on various treatments and ways to access them. We honored the dead through the creation of an evolving monument, the AIDS quilt.

And this terrible disease opened our hearts to love and an incredible, enduring sadness while we continued to go on. All this from a community of people who had come to exist as a community a mere fifteen to twenty years ago.

With the advent of AIDS funding, the lesbian/gay community suddenly found itself running multi-million dollar organizations, and an AIDS establishment was built. The AIDS/ARC crisis and its ensuing organizations became the lesbian/gay movement, and nearly all other issues took second stage. Indeed, the leaders of the AIDS establishment became the leaders of the lesbian/gay movement, some of whom were not even lesbians or gay men, but experts in AIDS. Not surprisingly, AIDS took priority over all our other needs as lesbians and gay men. Since the crisis was building rapidly and the need to respond was immediate, there was little analysis of the implications of our choices and actions. Where the money came from or the caveats for its use were issues rarely addressed, and connections to deficiencies in the health and social service systems affecting the larger community were generally ignored.

Response to the AIDS crisis has had an enormous impact on lesbians. Many of us involved in the women's movement turned our attentions to the lesbian/gay movement. There were many reasons for this shift. AIDS is a clear, delineated crisis, and there is an urgent need to help people in our community. Women, even lesbians, were raised to be caregivers in general and caregivers to men in particular. And even though lesbians have made a conscious choice to disown that heritage, we have nonetheless incorporated many of its basic tenets.

While there have always been unaddressed and painful divisions between lesbians and gay men, coming to the service of men around the issue of AIDS served finally to validate our existence. We could work with relative safety because by and large, we don't get AIDS, our lovers won't get AIDS, nor will our lesbian neighbors. We can even, sometimes, work in a queer environment. The work structures are set out for us; the funding is available. And AIDS is something the whole society is addressing; we can actually fit in, be considered heroic, important, decent, and be recognized for it. We get to work where our hearts lie.

This is not to say that working in AIDS is easy, or that we don't care about the people we know with AIDS. It is to say that we are making excruciating choices without even being aware of them.

While the women's movement still pulses with creativity and excitement, many of the institutions, services, and political agendas have disappeared. No one takes care of women or lesbians except women or lesbians, and we have a hard time taking care of ourselves, of finding ourselves worthy and important enough for attention. We are told that the process of change is a slow and plodding one. But we know that only when concerns are taken seriously does action follow.

As a woman with cancer, I have had to come face to face with how serious the situation is for women with cancer in our community; I have had to learn about what we need and what we don't have—the hard way. When I was waiting for my first biopsy result in May of 1985, I remember sitting in a Lesbian/Gay Advisory Committee meeting of the San Francisco Human Rights Commission. Our meeting focused on AIDS, and I remember thinking—screaming internally, really—what about me?

I had a lumpectomy followed by radiation. I survived, and was expected to go back to my life and my work, to work on AIDS.

If you have AIDS, you can go to the AIDS Foundation for food and social services advocacy; you can receive emergency funding through the AIDS Emergency Fund; you can get excellent meals through Project Open Hand. Your animals are taken care of should you land in the hospital or become too sick to care for them yourself. There are clinics, alternative centers, and organizations fighting for drugs and research and mental health needs of people with AIDS.

But if you have cancer, you wait endlessly for a support group. And if you are a lesbian, a woman of color, working class, and/or believe in alternative approaches to treating cancer, you don't fit into the few groups that are available. No organization shepherds you through the social service maze. No group brings you luscious meals or sends support people to clean your house or hold your hand.

Ignoring the needs of people with cancer is more typical of our culture. We live in a society which by and large does not take care of its sick. When people in our community suffer pain and deprivation, hardly anyone seems to give a damn. In the case of AIDS, however, we have—as a community—built a model of social response to a crisis, but a model which has not been replicated outside of AIDS.

Cancer, like AIDS, is about living. It's about living with a life-threatening disease, in whatever state, in whatever condition. As an activist, I have learned that action and change take place through collective support. My own cancer experience has strengthened my belief that all disease and illness are not only physiological, but also political.

I took some of what I learned in AIDS work and much of what I learned from feminist organizing and women's liberation, and together with other women created the Women's Cancer Resource Center. We desperately needed a resource, support, and advocacy center where women with cancer could be empowered to make their own choices and be supported by other women—a center controlled by women with cancer. I knew this vision was possible because the models had already been built for AIDS, as well as in the women's community.

The Women's Cancer Resource Center (WCRC) has been slow to grow, partly because some of us who have, or have had, cancer need to spend most of our energies taking care of our health. Many women are no longer involved in organizing work, but instead have turned their energies into working solely on themselves. Most of the remaining activists' energy is going into the fight against AIDS. Further, the WCRC is not in the closet about having lesbians on the advisory committee, nor—though we are an agency which serves all women with cancer—are we quiet about offering services to lesbians. Consequently, the homophobia of our society prevents us from receiving much in the way of funding, and those funding agencies which are not deterred by homophobia consider that they have sufficiently funded efforts on behalf of lesbian/gay people when they give money to AIDS projects.

Even with all these obstacles, WCRC has blossomed and flourished. The advisory committee worked on funding and programming; we began a drop-in support group; we presented forums and educationals; we started information sources on referrals and counseling; we produced successful fundraisers; we found and organized an office from which we can work and into which we can welcome all women with cancer who need help and support.

Then I found another lump in my breast. There were further tests, revealing that the cancer had spread to my lungs and bones. I could not believe that I was so ill. I had been exercising, feeling great, working long hours just as I had before the initial diagnosis. Despite my shock, however, I was not really surprised. Somehow I knew; I understood the precariousness of good health. Cancer had never been that far from my mind. And now, here it was again. For a time I fell apart, knowing the implications of this spread, knowing women who had metastatic breast cancer, knowing women who had died.

Finally I made my decisions. I used what I had learned over the past three years as a cancer activist and also what I had learned as an AIDS activist and feminist. I agonized over every choice as I went through my treatments and did my research. But I lived with a great deal of support from my lover, Teya, and from friends and acquaintances. These people I love. I cannot always express the extent of that love, but it is very present, and it gives me extreme pleasure as well as extreme pain.

One evening at my house, for instance, my acupuncturist was giving me treatment, a friend had gone food shopping and was putting the food away, a third friend was washing vegetables for juicing, and still another had just brought me a macrobiotic meal. The feelings of love I had for these people were indescribable, but at the same I time I wished my friends weren't there. I wished they could be doing something else, that they were not there because I needed them so much. With the first diagnosis, my life's axis permanently tilted; with this diagnosis, I live constantly on the edge.

But we who must battle cancer need more than our friends. We need knowledge and resources. Just as we were women and experts in our fields in the Middle Ages, so we need to lay claim to our heritage now. We have many people in nascent stages of expertise, but not enough experts. When we started the women's health movement, we began by taking control of our reproductive and gynecological health care. Now we need specialists in cancer, lupus, arthritis, environmental illness. We need practitioners in allopathic medicine, Chinese medicine, homeopathy, chiropractic. Lesbians can't afford to go to a "regular" doctor hoping for someone who is not homophobic. An oncology nurse at a recent forum on women and cancer reminded us that just because doctors have become aware of gay men due to AIDS, we can't assume they are less homophobic when they deal with lesbians. We need practitioners who are experts in their fields and clinics which are supportive of us as lesbians.

When lesbians get sick, we also get poor. Women are on a low rung of the financial ladder, and when we become ill, the bottom falls out much quicker because we are closer to it. We lose our health insurance and can't get more. If we are lucky enough to have a job, we have to stay in it. Many women I know work in situations where working feels almost physically unbearable because they can't afford to do anything else. Some of us who are unemployed would love to work, but no one will hire us. Some of us who are sick receive SSI payments but are hardly making it since, cruelly, the amount is so low.

One of the reasons that AIDS has become "different" from other diseases is because of the community organizing around it. Although diseases such as cancer have not yet had that kind of organized community support, we need to examine the information we are given about cancer with an eye towards its politics. There are politics in everything.

Cancer has had the American Cancer Society controlling information about the disease and controlling all the resources in the fight against it. The people on the board of the American Cancer Society, as well as other cancer institutions, are people with a lot of power in this society—power to maintain the status quo, thereby keeping themselves in power. Often they are representatives of chemical and pharmaceutical companies and the very scientists who stand to gain wealth and power from cancer research, and that research is geared to big bucks, not to actual prevention.

Real prevention would mean changing fundamental social structures. It would mean going after the tobacco industry, stopping the pollution of our environment, providing quality food. But when the medical profession talks about prevention, they mean at best small, individual acts—like stopping smoking and reducing dietary fat intake. When they talk about prevention, they talk about early detection methods like mammograms or breast self-examination. But once a tumor is found in your breast, you already have cancer, raising the question about whether early detection actually lengthens survival rates or simply lengthens the time you know you have cancer.

When a study came out a few years ago asserting that breast self-examination was meaningless,[6] I was furious. Most women I knew with breast cancer had found their cancer through breast exams. When doctors talk about early detection and admonish patients for not coming in sooner, they imply that an earlier appointment might have meant a cure would have been possible. Yet many women walk around with lumps in their breasts for a long time and go from doctor to doctor being repeatedly told that it's nothing, that it's "just fibrocystic breasts," that they will "watch it." I have known women who died fairly quickly after a diagnosis of breast cancer because their concerns about lumps in their breasts were ignored by doctors, and they were able to get attention only when their cancer had become quite advanced.

Groups facing health crises are often pitted against each other, and it is important for us to understand the reasons for those divisions. Many people with cancer are upset about the attention paid to AIDS. This inequality is not the fault of the people with AIDS, but rather of the systems that create the divisions. People start fighting over the same piece of the pie. It is not an accident.

Recently there was a report in the press about the AIDS crisis decimating funding for the National Cancer Institute, as the money was being taken from cancer research and going to AIDS. It wasn't taken from the military budget or the space budget. So the researchers in various diseases compete with each other, and consequently people who have the diseases do the same thing. Government and corporate researchers not only have not found a cure for cancer, but they continue to allow its spread while remaining apparently unwilling to offer adequate services to people who have cancer.

We need money for both cancer and AIDS. And we need a National Cancer Institute that does relevant research, not research into a quick cure that costs a fortune. Instead we need real prevention, real cure. We all know that pollution causes cancer, but the NCI and the American Cancer Society do nothing about the root causes of this disease. Just as we question what is said about AIDS, we need to question what is said about cancer, or any other disease.

Earlier in the women's movement, we took what had victimized us—rape, battery, incest—and worked toward changing society while making ourselves stronger. Now we tend to work only on ourselves individually; we do not make connections to the world, nor do we see that the world should change. Much of our energy is now put into therapy work, but without changing the environment which fosters victimization, that exploitation is allowed to continue. In that vein, a new disease model has emerged which holds that the individual is responsible for her illness.

We are a culture obsessed with looks and with health. The sort of thinking exemplified by the fitness craze rests on a faulty premise—the postulate that one's health is totally within the control of the individual. This premise presupposes that we create our own reality and that we have ultimate freedom of choice and total control over our own destinies.

When I first got out of the hospital, I opened a gay newspaper to find a positive review of a book called *The Silent Wound*.[7] The book was about how women get breast cancer because of repressed sexuality and conflicting new roles. Just like intellectuals get brain cancer? But beyond the nonsense put forth in the book, what really angered me was that a progressive newspaper in our community was lauding such nonsense as being enlightened, when all it did was feed into the notion of women's passivity and the individualization and psychological basis of disease.

I cannot count the number of people who have told me that I must not have had a positive attitude, for if I had I would not have gotten cancer. This pronouncement is cruel. I have also been told never to get angry because anger, too, is bad. I have been told that I worked too hard, thereby taking too much stress upon myself. Such thinking reflects a society which does not want us to be angry, which does not want us to be activists. We need to resist this sort of tranquilizer; instead, we need to ask why our culture wants to lull us into submission.

Not only do we fall prey to the emotional-causation nonsense, we are told that faulty spirituality causes cancer. The Puritans used to think that money was a sign of God's grace, and now we have come to think that health is such a sign. We have courses in miracles and karma, showing us, if we are ill, that something we have done in the past is causing our troubles now; we are working out our karma . . . what goes around comes around. Is that why women are raped and black people lynched? Karma? Such beliefs take the onus off the perpetrator, allow us to accept the unacceptable, forgive the unforgivable.

We have also romanticized death. Death is not lovely, not easy, most often not wanted. Romanticizing death makes it acceptable and welcome. We are excused from the struggle against wrongful death from a rotting planet and a society which has its priorities turned around.

We live in a world with acid rain, with a hole in the ozone layer, where food is mass produced and picked early with no nutrients, where pesticides are sprayed on the workers and the food we eat, where the animals we eat are raised in a tortured environment and fed hormones and antibiotics. We live in a world that has chemical dumps under housing tracts, schools, and playgrounds. We live in a society that has nuclear reactors and nuclear dumps and nuclear waste and nuclear bombs that go off over us and underground, where winds spread the invisible molecules and atoms everywhere. We call it pollution. It is invisible violence.

Society must change and redirect itself to be life-affirming, where welfare and health care are respected, where profits don't count more than people, where we are free of chemical and radiation hazards, where good food is available, where each person is recognized as significant and worthy of life.

As women, we need to see ourselves again as healers. We need to see the interconnections of all these issues, to take the skills we have learned as feminists and apply them to our work in AIDS and our work with women. And then take the skills we have gotten from working in AIDS and apply them to women's health care. Let's bring it back home.

I have wondered whether the urgency I feel comes from the fact that I have cancer. But I think that my cancer has only served to bring my sense of urgency closer to me. I firmly believe that we are on the brink of disaster, and that we must be very forceful if we are to stop the destruction before there is no "us." We have to stop being nice girls and start fighting as though our lives depended on it. Because they do.

Editor's Note: This article is adapted from a speech given as the keynote address to the Lesbian Caregivers and the AIDS Epidemic Conference, January, 1989.

NOTES

1. Ginsburg, Marsha, "More Women Battle AIDS," *San Francisco Chronicle*, January 1, 1989, pp. A1, A20.
2. Austin Donald F., M.D., *Cancer in California: Cancer Incidence Rates for the San Francisco-Oakland Metropolitan Statistical Area 1980-1984, Technical Report No. 1,* Cancer Prevention Section and California Tumor Registry, California Department of Health Services, p. 6. Figures are adapted for 1988.
3. Ehrenreich, Barbara, and Deirdre English, *Witches, Midwives and Nurses: A History of Women Healers,* Feminist Press, Old Westbury, New York, 1973, p. 15.
4. Boston Women's Health Book Collective, *The New Our Bodies, Ourselves,* Simon & Schuster, Inc., New York, 1984, pp. 308-309.
5. Ehrenreich and English, p. 19.
6. "Study Questions Self-Exams for Breast Cancer," *San Francisco Chronicle*, April 24, 1987, p. 1.
7. Boyd, Peggy, *The Silent Wound,* Addison-Wesley, Reading, Massachusetts, 1984.

From the Trenches

LINDA REYES
as told to Judith Brady

People with cancer live in a different world from people who are well. Because there is no absolute cure for cancer, many of us who have it are caught in overwhelming emotional turmoil. We turn to our family and friends to bail us out, and there is no way they can carry this burden. They, too, are having to come to terms with their own losses as well as with what has happened to us.

Other people rarely recognize how defenseless cancer patients are, especially those who are very sick. Nor do we have easily available ways in this society to respond to those more urgent needs. All that most people with cancer have to count on is each other. That's why it will be people with cancer who take the leadership in challenging the cancer establishment by dragging cancer out into the open as a social and political issue, and that's why support groups are indispensable for us.

I came out of my first support group meeting feeling as though I'd been released from a very lonely prison. The emotional strength we can give each other is one of the most important aspects of group support. Most people I know who have cancer have also learned that it helps a lot to be armed with encouragement and information when we have to make our ways through the medical mazes and the social services labyrinths. But what happened recently to a woman in my support group is a good example of how vulnerable people who are really sick can be and how important a support group is.

Patricia is quite sick; she has been fighting breast cancer metastasized to her bones for years. Despite all the radiation, chemotherapy, and steroid/hormone therapy she has endured, there are newly active tumors all over her bones, and she's in a lot of pain most of the time. She has to take morphine to control the pain. One night not long ago, she realized that she had run out of one of the chemotherapeutic drugs she is taking, and she called the office of her doctor, who practices with a group of oncologists. It took several calls, but she finally got through the answering service to the doctor on call that night. She recognized his name as one of the partners, but he was not her regular physician. He questioned her about her drugs, and he immediately protested that he could not understand why her doctor would have prescribed MS Contin (a trade name for morphine) for her along with the chemotherapeutic drug she needed. MS Contin, he vehemently insisted, was definitely contraindicated if a patient was taking the drug for which she was asking. He told her that he certainly could not give her another prescription for that drug unless she surrendered to him her supply of MS Contin. He said that he would send over a messenger to pick up her MS Contin, and then he would return to her by messenger a supply of the drug she needed along with Dilaudid (a trade name for hydromorphone, another potent narcotic), the drug he maintained she should be using for pain. After a lengthy discussion and much pressure, she agreed.

Shortly thereafter her doorbell rang, and the man on her doorstep said he had been sent by the doctor. She gave him her supply of MS Contin, along with the identification card required by her hospital pharmacy. Then she waited. After several hours had gone by, she called the hospital pharmacy. When the pharmacist heard her story, he said to her, "Lady, you'd better call the police."

The policewoman who interviewed her told her that they had received fifteen calls that night with identical stories from patients of that particular oncology practice. It's likely that someone who worked for the answering service is behind this cruel racket. It's also likely that the other fourteen victims are not members of a support group, and it's my guess that they are probably in very precarious positions.

Patricia's family and friends mean well, but there is nearly always an element of denial in people who don't have cancer, and—like most of us—Patricia undoubtedly works to cushion them from the harsh reality. She knows she can level with the members of her support group, however, because we have worked to build a sense of trust among us. She can talk to us, knowing we will understand all the implications of this horrible experience.

I worry about the other fourteen people. The police can only advise them on how to protect themselves. If they do not have support groups, to whom can they turn?

I've never been the victim of such an unscrupulous crime, but my cancer support group has been incredibly important to me, even though I didn't find the group until I had been ill for seven years. I had had a mastectomy followed by more than five years with no recurrence. Then a tumor appeared in my remaining breast, and a year after that breast was surgically removed, the cancer spread to my lungs and bone, and I started a heavy chemotherapy regime.

During that time my husband and kids were wonderful. I could always count on them to take care of things when I felt rotten. But they couldn't really understand or help me deal with what I was going through, so I couldn't talk to them about my apprehensions. I knew that a support group would have been helpful, but I just couldn't find one, and when I got really sick I stopped looking because I no longer had the energy. My doctor finally told me about the Cancer Support Community.

By this time I'd already come through the worst of my cancer treatment and I'd been struggling by myself for a long time. Still, I knew that this disease was not over for me, and I knew that I needed to be around other people who had cancer. For one thing, I believed (and I still do) that I will die from cancer, and I could never talk with my family about my battle to accept death because it upset them too much. But I could talk to other people with the disease.

The group was also a place for me to contribute some of what I had learned during my years of struggling by myself. I really needed to share my knowledge, because being able to offer what I had learned to other people who have cancer made the long, lonely struggle worthwhile. One simple trick I learned, for instance, was how to deal with nausea by eating the right foods in the right amounts at the right times so I wouldn't vomit after chemotherapy treatments. I know that most doctors don't know these tricks, and I've never seen them written anywhere. I also learned that eating a special diet which was very high in protein and calories protected my body from the toxic effects of chemo drugs. My blood counts stayed high, I rarely succumbed to colds or flu, my vital organs stayed healthy, and my hair grew back within three months. I could share that knowledge with other people who were undergoing chemo.

When I finally found it, the support group was a great relief to me. I very quickly developed a closeness to the people in the group. Because we are often met with fear and evasion by others, people with cancer feel separate from the rest of the population, and we become almost like relatives to each other. In some ways we're like soldiers in a war who develop extremely close relationships while they are in the trenches. Veterans of those trenches who have received medals of honor have said that it wasn't bravery which led them to their courageous acts—it was an overpowering concern for the other soldiers with them in those trenches.

Like those soldiers who could not escape the roar of enemy fire, if you've got cancer you've got to accept the fact that you have an extremely dangerous, and possibly terminal, disease. Any degree of denial negates what emotional support is there to be had, and denying the threat of cancer also invalidates the experience of the other group members, those who have been grappling with the knowledge that they are seriously ill and that their disease may kill them.

There is every reason to be afraid of breast cancer—or any cancer. Cancer is a killer. People who won't face that fact can cause real problems in support groups. Such people have often spent their lives controlling, and their control has always worked before. But it won't work for cancer. They misuse the very good advice that the patient be partners with the doctor when they decide that they can control their lives—and their cancer—by avoiding the recommended treatment, or further, by avoiding the very fact that they have cancer. They think they are going to "put cancer in its place." Chemotherapy and radiation, or any of the alternative therapies, certainly interfere dramatically with one's usual routines, and the people who try to deny cancer try to control the disease by not changing their lifestyles or their habits at all. They take the "out of sight, out of mind" adage one step further to "out of mind, out of body."

One woman, who earned her living as a corporate management consultant, presented us with such a problem. She announced that she had told her doctor she was going to stop chemotherapy. She had tumors in her lungs and had been treated with a mild chemotherapy regimen which hadn't worked. The only thing the doctors could do to prolong her life was offer aggressive chemotherapy, but she felt that would interfere with her lifestyle. She was self-employed and couldn't afford the changes chemo would make, she said. Two of us tried to get her to re-examine this judgment. She was adamant, however. She wanted the group to rubber-stamp her choice to believe that she could control her disease. The group couldn't do it, and she declared that maybe we weren't the group for her if we couldn't support whatever decision she made.

Although she stayed in the group, we never again put our knowledge and our feelings on the line for her. Within six months the cancer metastasized to her brain. She's now dead. No one can say that aggressive chemotherapy would have saved her, but she was not willing to give it a chance, not willing to face the very real threat to her life. Cancer is a swift-moving, unpredictable disease.

That woman's decision to ignore her cancer was different from deciding to try an alternative approach. Had she decided that she would undergo an alternative treatment—whatever it might have been—we would have supported her choice and done whatever we could to help her carry it through. Such a choice at least recognizes that cancer isn't like a cold which will eventually go away even if you ignore it.

Another woman I know vacillated over the decision to follow her doctor's recommendation that she have chemotherapy because she didn't know if having chemotherapy was "politically correct." She knew it was necessary for cancer patients to take an active role in deciding how they will treat their cancer, but whatever crowd she traveled with—and she called herself a feminist—had her so scared that the medical profession would undercut her autonomy that she would meaninglessly risk her life.

In truth, I wasn't much different. Before I ever had a diagnosis of breast cancer, I remember reading about it and about chemotherapy. Being nearly phobic about nausea and stomachaches, I thought to myself that if I ever had breast cancer, I would never consent to that modern chamber of horrors known as chemotherapy—I would instead do the Simonton visualization.* But then when I did get breast cancer, I was much too angry to do any visualization. My original diagnosis was border-

* The Simonton program, developed by Dr. O. Carl Simonton and Stephanie Simonton-Atchley while they were practicing in Fort Worth, Texas, is an intensive group psychotherapy program which includes visualization and is designed to facilitate treatment already being received by the patient. The Simonton Cancer Center is in Pacific Palisades, California.

line Stage II breast cancer, and the doctor gave me a choice of whether or not to do chemotherapy. I absolutely refused it.

Who knows whether I was right or wrong. Who knows whether a different conclusion would have made a difference in the course of my disease. The point is that I was not making a decision. I was reacting emotionally. Had I been in a support group, I might instead have made a rational decision because I would have had a place to thrash it all out. I might in the end have decided no to the chemotherapy, but that refusal would have been a considered no, not just an emotional and fearful no.

By the third meeting of the group, I had a really urgent need for their support, because my husband had just been diagnosed with lung cancer. I actually knew about Tom's diagnosis a week before I was able to talk about it. My world nearly collapsed when I learned that he had this very dangerous cancer with a very poor prognosis. Tom had been my only personal support system for years. He was my financial support, too, and I was going to lose this, though I don't think this fear surfaced for a while. Mostly I was simply overwhelmed that somebody I loved had gotten this terrible disease.

I'm not a person who can easily show emotion in public. The last time I had cried in front of other people, I was six years old. But the support group had already built in me the trust I needed to tell them what had happened, and that trust also gave me the permission I needed to cry. It was a healing cry; all the grief was allowed to come out. And I could do it because I felt so very close to each person in that room.

Tom was sick for more than a year before he died. My children helped me manage most of the caring for him, but during that time the support group really held me together. They also offered me practical aid; one woman came and stayed with Tom a few times so that I could do errands.

Tom has been dead for two years now, and I have survived cancer for ten years. My cancer support group is still as important to me as ever. Since Tom's death I have had many, many new battles to face, and the support group has given me the strength to do it. Just because we are people with cancer, that is not the only problem we have to deal with, and cancer is not all that we can talk about in the group. We discuss many other parts of our lives, just as more traditional therapy groups do. Yet for me as a woman with cancer, there is a need to talk about those other aspects of my life with people who understand me as a person with cancer. Even if the cancer is not at this particular moment my most urgent situation, for me there is always—as there is for all of us—the nagging fear that any other problems we are handling just might activate the cancer. People who have not faced cancer just can't understand that fear.

Death from this disease is part of the reality we have to face. Some people have left the group because other members have died. I've been through a lot of deaths in two different support groups to which I've belonged. I had thought about this aspect of becoming intimate with other cancer patients before I first joined a group, and I had decided that I could handle it. The deaths which were the most difficult for me were the young deaths. Ava, thirty-two, a pediatrician with so much to give—I still grieve for Ava. Yet I have never wanted to leave because people died, though I've seen other group members decide to leave because they couldn't handle it. Like too many doctors who counsel their cancer patients not to join support groups, those people thought of death as only negative, and they seemed to feel that if they walked away from that negativity they would be walking toward health. These people made the mistake of seeing everybody else's death as their own. I never did that; in fact, I find that sort of identification a bit offensive. A person's birth and life are his or her own, and so is his or her death—you cannot take it from them.

My battle in the trenches took a new turn a year after Tom's death. I learned that there was a new group starting at the Cancer Support Community for women with metastatic breast cancer. A number of women who were members of more general cancer support groups and who had metastatic breast disease had asked for a support group of their own, because the issues which they had to deal with were different from and often more urgent than those of people with newly diagnosed cancers. I was asked to chair the first meeting of the group because I was familiar with support group dynamics and because I had been fighting metastatic breast cancer for a number of years. One of the first strategic decisions we made was to meet weekly. Slowly, we've built up a solid group. I think, for me, my early success of keeping this new group alive by following up on it, by keeping in touch with people and pushing them to keep coming, primed me for more action.

One of the women who became part of the group was from New York. At an early meeting she burst out, "What is *wrong* with you women in the Bay Area? Where's your political savvy? There are no groups to fight breast cancer out here at all!"

And so the idea was born. Another woman in that support group was also interested in the educational and political aspects of breast cancer, and she became the president of our new organization, Breast Cancer Action (BCA). I wanted to help start an organization which would devote itself to getting out the real facts about breast cancer. I wanted the whole nation to know what was really happening with breast cancer: forty years of no effective prevention had caused the incidence of breast cancer to spiral to epidemic proportions. Worst of all, it was now moving rapidly down the generational ladder to women in their thirties and late twenties. I wanted information spread through every available source so that every woman in this country could know what was going on and know what she could do if she were unlucky enough to be the one out of nine women in this country who hear the diagnosis of breast cancer. We all have to know; none of us can remain deaf and dumb about what is happening to women—this year more than 44,500 will die from this disease and next year it will probably be more. Those projections are a blasphemy in my mind.

We're organizing at a good time. Recently, there have been quite a few articles in major publications.* We've received telephone calls from all over the country from women who want to know how to start political action groups like ours.

Breast Cancer Action has established its aims. Within the framework of the primary goal, which is to abolish breast cancer, we seek:

1. An end to the biases of gender and age in medical research and treatment;

---

* For instance, an article by Jane Gross, "Turning Disease Into a Cause: Breast Cancer Follows AIDS" appeared in the January 7, 1991 issue of *The New York Times*; "The Politics of Breast Cancer" by Melinda Beck et al. appeared in the December 10, 1990 issue of *Newsweek*, and "A Puzzling Plague" by Claudia Wallis was a cover story in the January 14, 1991 issue of *Time* magazine.

2. A demonstrable willingness to uncover the causes of breast cancer, whether environmental, dietary, or whatever and wherever it takes the government, research community, and all segments of society;

3. Significantly increased legislative and financial support for treatment research to move toward a cure;

4. Access to information—from doctors, drug companies, and government agencies;

5. Serious, considered response to our questions regarding the decisions of the Food and Drug Administration, the National Cancer Institute, the American Cancer Society, and the American Medical Association;

6. A social framework in which breast cancer is a sociopolitical public health issue, not a personal tragedy. This includes the involvement and support of well people, and men as well as women;

7. Emotional support of women with breast cancer regarding such issues as body image, hair loss, sexuality, family concerns, job issues, as well as sickness and dying;

8. In the short term, insurance coverage for new treatments which have demonstrated efficacy but may still be under investigation;

9. In the long term, access to affordable, competent health care for everyone.

One of our aims is to make connections with all the other cancer organizations out there so we can work together. We are interested, for instance, in the Breast Cancer Centers in Sweden which came into being because Swedish women demanded them. The Centers sound wonderful. Unlike our situation in this country, all the mammogram machines in the Swedish centers are regulated and the operators well trained. Kaiser Permanente, a Health Maintenance Organization with various facilities on the West Coast, has imported Swedish technicians to teach their technicians. In Sweden, if a woman is called back after a mammogram, another mammogram is done along with a sonogram. All follow-up happens within this one center, and the centers are spread all throughout the country. If the woman has cancer, she is given her options and the team's appraisal of her condition. Here, if a woman has more than one doctor, the different physicians seldom even know each other.

We have much to learn from Sweden. But a priority now has to be getting the word out. There are too many places in the United States where women have no resources to turn to when they hear the diagnosis of cancer. We in BCA want to help women set up support groups; it's not difficult to do and you don't need an "expert." There are not nearly enough support groups around. Over the past few years, I've become a sort of telephone counselor because other people I know send people they know who have cancer to me. A woman just called me from Vacaville; there are no support groups anywhere near her. Another woman from Half Moon Bay called, and it was the same story with her: no support groups near her.

We also want to help women set up political action groups like ours. BCA is different from a support group. As a political action group, we need people with energy and stamina, and many people with cancer just don't have either. So we have some healthy women in BCA—that makes it different from support groups where healthy women would be inappropriate. Healthy women in BCA not only give the organization more physical and emotional energy, they also make it clear to other healthy women that breast cancer is not an issue which they should avoid.

We've learned a lot from our time in the trenches. We've had to stay in those ditches because we were too few and too weak to wage all-out war from every possible vantage point. But as more and more of us become seasoned veterans in this war against cancer, there will be so many of us that we can no longer stay in those trenches. Then the battle against cancer will at last be ours to fight and maybe even someday to win.

Finding Community

BEVERLY ROSS
as told to Mary Ryan

Hearing the diagnosis of cancer can be a pretty devastating experience. From that point on, things don't usually get much better, and for most of us it's very hard to ask for help from friends or family or even from lovers. In that respect, I was lucky, because when I heard that diagnosis I could turn to the Mautner Project for Lesbians with Cancer.

The Mautner Project opened its doors in Washington, D.C. in January of 1990. It began as the vision of Mary-Helen Mautner, a lesbian lawyer who was diagnosed with breast cancer in 1982 and had a a recurrence in 1986. Three weeks before she died in August of 1989, Mary-Helen Mautner wrote, and left to her partner, Susan Hester, a page of notes about an idea for a project for lesbians who have life-threatening illnesses. People were asked to donate to such a project as a memorial to Mary-Helen. A few months after Mary-Helen's death, Susan Hester called a meeting. Twenty-five women showed up. By the second meeting, people agreed that the project should focus on cancer and on the needs of lesbians with the disease.

Only a few weeks before that first meeting was called, I was basking in the warmth of a new love and reveling in the afterglow of a birthday party which had attracted forty friends and left me feeling appreciated and joyful. Finally, my life seemed to be coming together. I had a job I enjoyed, good friends, my health, and high hopes. And best of all, I was madly in love with Linda.

Then one day I did a breast self-examination. This time something was different. There was a mass, large and soft, under the left nipple. A quick check confirmed my suspicions; my right breast was its usual smooth, fat, soft self. I wasn't too worried. Breast lumps are common and most are benign. Besides, this lump didn't feel anything like the ones in the silicone demonstration breasts at the Health Fair. But cancer is a disease for which I have a lot of respect, so I promptly scheduled a visit with my doctor.

It was cancer. I was disappointed, of course, that the lump was malignant, but I felt fortunate that we'd caught it at the earliest stage. After all the treatment options had been explained, I elected to have a mastectomy. The surgery went well, thanks not only to the medical people, but also to a wonderful group of friends. Linda was with me as I went into surgery, and she was there when I woke up. I emerged from the hospital flat-chested on one side with a big, nasty scar running from my sternum to my armpit and a truly icky drain hanging out of my side. Thanks to Linda, the ugliness never got the better of me.

At this point the Mautner Project entered my life. The first organizational meeting was to be held the day before I returned to work. When I heard about it, I knew I had to go; this wasn't just a coincidence—it was an opportunity.

After the first community meeting I wasn't sure how I would fit in. Though not all of the women at that first meeting had cancer or a partner with cancer, the sick people were, by and large, sicker than I was. Further, most of the women there were feminists who were veterans of all sorts of early struggles, and I had barely been involved in any sort of women's organization. And the women there were so open about being lesbians that I assumed they had been out of the closet for a long time, while I was just beginning to recognize that I was a lesbian and just beginning to talk about my identity.

It was a wonderful group of women. I was surprised and moved that some there did not have cancer but simply wanted to do something positive for the lesbian community in the D.C. area. I came home from that first meeting so high! It was several days before it hit me that some of these great women were very sick and some were going to die. I went from being very high to very low, and then came back again to a renewed acceptance of my own mortality.

During that first meeting, the Project established four main avenues of activity:

1. Biweekly support groups;
2. Direct services for lesbians with cancer, their partners, families and caregivers;
3. Education about cancer to the lesbian community;
4. Information to the health care community about the needs of lesbians with cancer.

We divided into four work groups to brainstorm ideas about how we could accomplish each of these tasks. By the end of that first meeting, we had a mailing list and volunteers to take care it. I had found my niche. I would be coming back.

Since that first meeting the Mautner Project established a variety of working groups which meet during the month and report back to the general membership. The support group for lesbians with cancer, their partners and caregivers was one of the first Project groups to get started. My partner and I volunteered to facilitate the support group, which meets twice a month.

All of us in that group benefit from a sense of community. It's fairly easy to find a mainstream support group for people with cancer, and it's not too difficult to find a group of lesbians. But to find a group of people who understand being a lesbian *and* having cancer is uniquely wonderful. Here I can be myself without explaining a lot of things. We share recovery and relapse, joy and disappointment. We talk about dying, we look at the ravages of chemotherapy, and we celebrate the joy of living for the moment.

We are buddies under fire, and we work as a family to be there for one another. I've found in this group the sisters I never had. When one of our members died I had to be willing to be in touch with my own fear, my own mortality. My reward for this struggle has been the company of women who are living courageously each day, striving to find the energy to go to work week after week while undergoing chemotherapy, deciding that this time a scarf will do instead of a wig. Their courage is contagious and puts me in touch with my own. If I ever have to face similar battles myself, I will know that others have been there before me and have done well.

The Mautner Project's direct services extend far beyond the support group. We provide logistical support in a variety of ways, from finding blood replacements to offering rides to the hospital for treatment. One volunteer arranges for child care, another does the grocery shopping, while still another took someone Christmas shopping. Often it is the little things that mean the most, by helping someone who is gravely ill maintain a sense of normalcy. Direct service volunteers will do just about any little chore that someone requests. A lesbian with cancer, her partner, or a friend can request a "buddy," and the direct service volunteer will do whatever she can to assist. Sometimes it is as simple as calling and "checking in" every couple of weeks or as complicated as putting together a team of volunteers to meet the needs of the woman with cancer and/or her partner. These volunteers are a very caring and supportive group of women.

The Project holds training sessions for anyone, not just the direct service volunteers, who would like to attend and participate in some way in the life of the Mautner Project. Those sessions impart a lot of information about cancer and how it affects a person's life, but they also function to build our community. They are times for all of us to come together, to hear each other's stories, and to know that we are all human and mortal.

Educational events are an important component of the Project. Lesbians are at higher risk for some cancers because fewer of us have children before the age of thirty, and many of us do not see a physician regularly, which can delay detection. A radiologist and a well-known breast cancer specialist lectured at our very first educational event, which attracted over 200 people. We've placed public service announcements in the local lesbian and gay newspapers to raise cancer awareness. We have produced a brochure for health care providers which explains the Mautner Project and includes Rolodex cards with information about the Project.

There are, of course, immediate political implications any time a group of women get together to form a health-oriented organization. Our health issues have been ignored by the medical establishment for a very long time, and the experiences which people in the support group have shared with us have raised our awareness of the enormous task before us. For instance, some women have had problems with health care providers who have difficulty recognizing our partners as our next of kin. We are developing a role for ourselves as advocates and hope to do in-service training at local hospitals.

I know this past year of work with the Mautner Project has changed me. I've learned a great deal from having a potentially fatal illness, and that's been very important. The whole year has been one of growth and of finding myself. My relationship with Linda has deepened and we are now "out" to our friends as a couple. I'm sure this would have happened eventually, but my illness and my involvement with this new community have speeded things up. I have much to thank the Project for, as do many others. But the Project is really us; it's nothing more than the shared vision of women caring for and supporting each other in the best ways we can.

I am very happy for us and also very proud of the Project. It seems nearly impossible that all this could have happened in only a year! So many members of our community, even women who have never been personally touched by this illness, have poured a tremendous amount of energy into the Project, and we have all benefited as a result. The mailing list has grown to more than 500 names, including more than 100 volunteers, and our first fundraising project was more successful than we expected. New women come to each general meeting and feel welcomed. We have set goals for our second year that are even more ambitious than the first year. There is life and excitement and a common purpose that all of us share. I truly have found community.

Challenging the Establishment

SUSAN LIROFF
as told to Ines Rieder and Frédérique Delacoste

The Women's Cancer Resource Center (WCRC), of which I am the director, is a staunchly independent organization. First established in 1986 by Jackie Winnow, the WCRC is located in a small, friendly office on Shattuck Avenue in Berkeley, California and provides a variety of services for women with cancer, their friends, families, health practitioners, and communities.

We have a small budget based on income from private donations, a few small grants and fundraising benefits. We pay one part-time staff person, but mostly we rely on volunteer labor to maintain all our services: legal, medical, and social service information and referral; support groups; peer counseling; advocacy; telephone hotline; community educational forums; speakers' bureau; classes in visualization, massage, nutrition, and stress reduction; and a library. We are always looking for volunteers not only to maintain our present activities, but also to develop strategies to extend our influence as one of the few feminist organizations in the United States dealing specifically with cancer-related women's issues. But ultimately we want and need to have paid staff, because the success of the health care movement depends on paid labor.

For the first two years of its existence, the WCRC was primarily a one-woman operation run by Jackie Winnow out of her home. Then three years ago Jackie's breast cancer metastasized, and she could no longer carry the lion's share of responsibility for WCRC. Shortly before Jackie learned of her recurrence, I had been diagnosed with breast cancer myself. By the time I was pretty well recovered from my surgery, Jackie told us that she might have to shut down the WCRC. I knew personally how important the center had been to me. I asked what I could do to keep it going.

I began taking on some of the work Jackie had been doing—writing letters, responding to telephone calls. But there was an obvious need for us to expand, so we called as many interested women as we could think of and asked them to come to a meeting. Fourteen women showed up. We started by trying to establish various committees, but somehow that never seemed to work. The energy just wasn't there to sustain separate committees. Finally, three or four women out of the original fourteen formed ourselves into one committee which took on the task of building the WCRC into the organization it has become. Right now we have a steering committee of nine women, seven of whom came to the WCRC because they have cancer. We serve primarily those women who are most likely to be neglected by existing programs: women of color, lesbians, older women, and low-income women.

A basic premise of this Center is that the responsibility for the disease does *not* lie with the individual who has cancer. We feel it is very important that our group leaders agree with that premise, and it's the first message we try to get across in our support groups. We do believe that it *is* up to us, however, once we have cancer, to decide how we will handle our lives. The Center—particularly through our support groups—provides a safe and reassuring community in which to make those decisions. We are not able to alter the ultimate course of our cancer as much as we would like; rather, our strength is in affecting the quality of our lives.

We try to provide as wide a range of resources and information as possible so that we can respond to all sorts of different requests, whether or not those requests reflect our philosophies. If a woman calls us to find out where she can get psychic healing to cure her cancer—not an approach we particularly support—we don't hang up on her; we give her some ideas about where to go.

Anybody can walk through the door and start working here. While we do not exclude any woman who needs our services or who wants to contribute to our work, we do discourage people who proselytize the New Age doctrine of self-blame or self-causation. We do not agree that certain attitudes, past antagonisms, or negative energies cause cancer. I would certainly invite someone with such an attitude to sit down at the computer and do data input for as long as she liked, but women with that perspective would never be charged with support group leadership.

We are very careful when choosing the women to lead our support groups. We run facilitator training sessions during which we spend the whole day in encounter situations, bringing out all the sensitive issues and seeing how people react. We have an ongoing facilitator team which meets regularly, and, at this point, we assume that women with philosophies which are antithetical to the outlook of this Center will quickly discover that this is not the place for them.

We are excited about being part of a patient/activist health care movement which is taking shape in the United States. We consider ourselves to be a consumer-based health organization which promotes peer support, counseling, and a general restructuring of the health care system. We are part of a movement which intends to confront the government about its twisted spending priorities. Women have been organizing around health issues for years, but certainly none of us who are in our thirties and forties ever expected that we would have to organize around cancer. The rates of breast cancer, for instance, for women in the age group of thirty-five to forty have tripled in the 1980s. We either have cancer ourselves or we know someone who has it. The AIDS movement opened a lot of eyes about community organizing around health issues, and now women are starting to see cancer as an important issue for us.

What brings many different kinds of women together in this organization is the fact that we have cancer or that cancer has intimately touched our lives because someone we know or love has been diagnosed with the disease. We have some radical lesbians and we have many women who would never have thought of going, for instance, to an International Women's Day march but who might consider doing so now. The WCRC has been around for four years now, writing, talking, putting on educational programs about cancer, and marching wherever we could with signs about cancer. I think it's interesting that we've exposed some conservative women to more progressive politics just by being involved in cancer issues. But because we are an activist Center, we have not attracted truly conservative women who would support other, more traditional sorts of cancer organizations.

In California, groups are forming to lobby for legislative relief and for more research money specifically for breast cancer. There is the Northern California Breast Cancer Organization, a coalition consisting of Breast Cancer Action in San Francisco, Save Our Selves in Sacramento, Y-Me Bay Area Breast Cancer Network in Saratoga, and most recently the WCRC.

We at the WCRC have some differences with these other groups because they limit the scope of attention to just breast cancer. It's certainly true that breast cancer is a major killer of women, but just recently we lost two women who were very close to our hearts to cervical cancer and Hodgkin's disease. They were both under forty. I think it would be a mistake for us to open the door to a financial or legislative "divide and conquer" routine—that is, the funding of research and/or resources for breast cancer only, excluding women who are stricken with other forms of the disease.

The National Cancer Institute (NCI) controls enormous amounts of money while totally ignoring the social and environmental questions concerning the epidemiology of cancer. They're still searching for individual solutions to, or cures for, the disease, spending the bulk of their time and resources in arguing over drugs. They certainly don't use their considerable clout to put any pressure on the food industry, for instance. Most American consumers apparently accept the idea that it is up to them individually to remain healthy; that line at least makes them feel they have some control. But all the advice which the NCI, or even the American Cancer Society (ACS), gives to consumers about how we should read labels before we buy food doesn't mean much to people who don't have the time to read those labels, or who can't read them, or who don't know the dangers of hydrogenated oils, for instance. The only real protection for consumers would come from forcing the food industries to stop putting stuff in the food that will poison us.

In the meantime, the Environmental Protection Agency has been effectively dismantled. We've not heard a word about that from either the National Cancer Institute or the American Cancer Society. As far as I know, none of these mainstream organizations has ever agitated for any meaningful changes. And that's why many hold them responsible for murder.

But even if the national headquarters of the ACS and Y-Me refuse to take real positions which might effect changes, it appears that their rank and file are showing signs of restlessness. They are starting to include breast cancer activism, in particular, on their agenda lest they be left in the dust. I think we'll be seeing lots of changes in terms of legislation and financial allocations for breast cancer and women's health in the near future, none of which would have come about if grassroots organizing had not taken place.

And there's a great deal more to be done on the grassroots level. For instance, we plan to begin weekly discussions on many different cancer-related topics, and we will have different people come in and speak. We want the WCRC to become a center for ongoing discussion and political dialogue between the women who are part of the center and all kinds of specialists. We want doctors and nurses to come and speak with us. We want to talk to alternative health care providers, environmental activists, legal advisors, and others working for community health care.

We've already begun meeting with members of the medical profession. A group of doctors from a local Health Maintenance Organization hospital recently asked us to come and meet with them. They wanted to know about the problems which women who come to the Center are having with them. We are in the process of establishing a liaison person to be at the hospital so that when we learn of any particular problems encountered by one of our members with that hospital, there is someone to call. One of the physicians who met with us is an instructor at the hospital, and he wanted our advice on how physicians should be trained. We raised a number of issues, among them the way that physicians ignore complaints and symptoms and accuse women of being hysterical when they insist they feel something which physicians apparently don't think they "should" be feeling.

We're also establishing a relationship with the county hospital, talking to their personnel about setting up a volunteer program to work with support groups at the in-patient and out-patient units within the hospital. At this point, the average life expectancy of someone who shows up at that county hospital with cancer is about six months. When people are finally forced to seek medical attention at the county hospital, usually their disease has already reached an advanced state. Most of the women who come to the county hospital are women of color.

It's been very gratifying to have this sort of interaction with the local medical community, though it's about time they recognize our role with their clients. We must be doing something right; we've certainly sent enough women to lawyers for the way their doctors dragged their heels. A few weeks ago we invited employees from the HMO, county hospitals, and a community health center which provides free screening to come and visit our Center. A lot of people came and several are going to return for our facilitator training. They will take back to their workplaces an understanding of not only our philosophy of empowerment, but also the importance of peer support.

Making connections with other local grassroots community organizations is another important aspect of our work. We're working with the Bay Area Black Women's Health Project. They are currently running our facilitator training. They've never before done this training around the issue of a specific health problem, like cancer, so our work with them makes the best use of our two areas of expertise. We know about cancer, and they know a great deal about group dynamics, how to establish a sense of trust and safety, how to approach a problem outside the constraints of professionalism. Any woman can be trained to be a facilitator—no one needs a degree.

We have really just begun. Nonetheless, our support is growing all the time. We recently did a fundraising mailing with faint hearts; we know the recession is on and that people have less discretionary money. But the response from the women's community was nothing short of amazing—it was the best response to a mailing that we've ever had. We got larger checks and pledges of monthly support from others who say that can't afford a large amount at one time. As times are getting harder, the women are coming through with more than ever.

The recent increase in media coverage is probably at least part of the reason for the very positive response to our fundraising. In the last month I've spent countless hours in interviews instead of getting the work done around here. The media exposure helps, however, not only to spread the word about the Center and organizing around the issue of cancer, but also to elicit funds from people who have read about our existence and our work. And we've had more women call to volunteer their time because they read about the Center.

As the director, I am primarily responsible for fundraising, for what we are able to do is largely dependent on how much money we have to spend doing it. We've had lots of discussions about where we should go to solicit funding; we don't want to have to adjust our ideas or our programs to suit any funders' restrictions, for example. Aside from that, I think every dime in this country is tainted, and it doesn't make too much difference where we get the money, though this is an area where we don't all agree. In any case, if organizations like the Women's Cancer Resource Center continue to spring up and grow in this country—as they seem to be doing—how we are funded will be less problematic, for the day might come when we hold the upper hand.

Selections from A Burst Of Light

AUDRE LORDE

November 8, 1986, New York City
　　If I am to put this all down in a way that is useful, I should start with the beginning of the story.

Sizable tumor in the right lobe of the liver, the doctors said. Lots of blood vessels in it means it's most likely malignant. Let's cut you open right now and see what we can do about it. Wait a minute, I said. I need to feel this thing out and see what's going on inside myself first, I said, needing some time to absorb the shock, time to assay the situation and not act out of panic. Not one of them said, I can respect that, but don't take too long about it.

Instead, that simple claim to my body's own processes elicited such an attack response from a reputable Specialist In Liver Tumors that my deepest—if not necessarily most useful—suspicions were totally aroused.

What the doctor could have said to me that I would have heard was, "You have a serious condition going on in your body and whatever you do about it you must not ignore it or delay deciding how you are going to deal with it because it will not go away no matter what you think it is." Acknowledging my responsibility for my own body. Instead, what he said to me was, "If you do not do exactly what I tell you to do right now without questions you are going to die a horrible death." In exactly those words.

I felt the battle lines being drawn up within my own body.

I saw this specialist in liver tumors at a leading cancer hospital in New York City, where I had been referred as an outpatient by my own doctor.

The first people who interviewed me in white coats from behind a computer were only interested in my health-care benefits and proposed method of payment. Those crucial facts determined what kind of plastic ID card I would be given, and without a plastic ID card, no one at all was allowed upstairs to see any doctor, as I was told by the uniformed, pistoled guards at all the stairwells.

From the moment I was ushered into the doctor's office and he saw my X-rays, he proceeded to infantalize me with an obviously well-practiced technique. When I told him I was having second thoughts about a liver biopsy, he glanced at my chart.

Racism and Sexism joined hands across his table as he saw I taught at a university. "Well, you look like an *intelligent girl*," he said, staring at my one breast all the time he was speaking. "Not to have this biopsy immediately is like sticking your head in the sand." Then he went on to say that he would not be responsible when I wound up one day screaming in agony in the corner of his office!

I asked this specialist in liver tumors about the dangers of a liver biopsy spreading an existing malignancy, or even encouraging it in a borderline tumor. He dismissed my concerns with a wave of his hand, saying, instead of answering, that I really did not have any other sensible choice.

I would like to think that this doctor was sincerely motivated by a desire for me to seek what he truly believed to be the only remedy for my sickening body, but my faith in that scenario is considerably diminished by his $250 consultation fee and his subsequent medical report to my own doctor containing numerous supposedly clinical observations of "obese abdomen" and "remaining pendulous breast."

In any event, I can thank him for the fierce shard lancing through my terror that shrieked there must be some other way, this doesn't feel right to me. If this is cancer and they cut me open to find out, what is stopping that intrusive action from spreading the cancer, or turning a questionable mass into an active malignancy? All I was asking for was the reassurance of a realistic answer to my real questions, and that was not forthcoming. I made up my mind that if I was going to die in agony on somebody's office floor, it certainly wasn't going to be his! I needed information, and pored over books on the liver in Barnes & Noble's Medical Textbook Section on Fifth Avenue for hours. I learned, among other things, that the liver is the largest, most complex, and most generous organ in the human body. But that did not help me very much.

In this period of physical weakness and psychic turmoil, I found myself going through an intricate inventory of rage. First of all at my breast surgeon—had he perhaps done something wrong? How could such a small breast tumor have metastasized? Hadn't he assured me he'd gotten it all, and what was this now anyway about micro-metastases? Could this tumor in my liver have been seeded at the same time as my breast cancer? There were so many unanswered questions, and too much that I just did not understand.

But my worst rage was the rage at myself. For a brief time I felt like a total failure. What had I been busting my ass doing these past six years if it wasn't living and loving and working to my utmost potential? And wasn't that all a guarantee supposed to keep exactly this kind of thing from ever happening again? So what had I done wrong and what was I going to have to pay for it and WHY ME?

But finally a little voice inside me said sharply, "Now really, is there any other way you would have preferred living the past six years that would have been more satisfying? And be that as it may, *should* or *shouldn't* isn't even the question. How do you want to live the rest of your life from now on and what are you going to do about it?" Time's awasting!

Gradually, in those hours in the stacks of Barnes & Noble, I felt myself shifting into another gear. My resolve strengthened as my panic lessened. Deep breathing, regularly. I'm not going to let them cut into my body again until I'm convinced there is no other alternative. And this time, the burden of proof rests with the doctors because their record of success with liver cancer is not so good that it would make me jump at a surgical solution. And scare tactics are not going to work. I have been scared now for six years and that hasn't stopped me. I've given myself plenty of practice in doing whatever I need to do, scared or not, so scare tactics are just not going to work. Or I hoped they were not going to work. At any rate, thank the goddess, they were not working yet. One step at a time.

But some of my nightmares were pure hell, and I started having trouble sleeping.

In writing this I have discovered how important some things are that I thought were unimportant. I discovered this by the high price they exact for scrutiny. At first I did not want to look again at how I slowly came to terms with my own mortality on a level deeper than before, nor with the inevitable strength that gave me as I started to get on with my life in actual time. Medical textbooks on the liver were fine, but there were appointments to be kept, and bills to pay, and decisions about my upcoming trip to Europe to be made. And what do I say to my children? Honesty has always been the bottom line between us, but did I really need them going through this with me during their final difficult years at college? On the other hand, how could I shut them out of this most important decision of my life?

I made a visit to my breast surgeon, a doctor with whom I have always been able to talk frankly, and it was from him that I got my first trustworthy and objective sense of timing. It was from him that I learned that the conventional forms of treatment for liver metastases made little more than one year's difference in the survival rate. I heard my old friend Clem's voice coming back to me through the dimness of thirty years: "I see you coming here trying to make sense where there is no sense. Try just living in it. Respond, alter, see what happens." I thought of the African way of perceiving life, as experience to be lived rather than as problem to be solved.

Homeopathic medicine calls cancer the cold disease. I understand that down to my bones that quake sometimes in their need for heat, for the sun, even for just a hot bath. Part of the way in which I am saving my own life is to refuse to submit my body to cold whenever possible.

In general, I fight hard to keep my treatment scene together in some coherent and serviceable way, integrated into my daily living and absolute. Forgetting is no excuse. It's as simple as one missed shot could make the difference between a quiescent malignancy and one that is growing again. This not only keeps me in an intimate, positive relationship to my own health, but it also underlines the fact that I have the responsibility for attending my own health. I cannot simply hand over that responsibility to anybody else.

Which does not mean I give in to the belief, arrogant or naive, that I know everything I need to know in order to make informed decisions about my body. But attending my own health, gaining enough information to help me understand and participate in the decisions made about my body by people who know more medicine than I do, are all crucial strategies in my battle for living. They also provide me with important prototypes for doing battle in all other arenas of my life.

Battling racism and battling heterosexism and battling apartheid share the same urgency inside me as battling cancer. None of these struggles are ever easy, and even the smallest victory is never to be taken for granted. Each victory must be applauded, because it is so easy not to battle at all, to just accept and call that acceptance inevitable.

November 10, 1986, New York City

Building into my living—without succumbing to it—an awareness of this reality of my life, that I have a condition within my body of which I will eventually die, comes in waves, like a rising tide. It exists side by side with another force inside me that says no you don't, not you, and the X-rays are wrong and the tests are wrong and the doctors are wrong.

There is a different kind of energy inherent within each one of these feelings, and I try to reconcile and use these different energies whenever I need them. The energy generated by the first awareness serves to urge me always to get on with living my life and doing my work with an intensity and purpose of the urgent now. Throw the toys overboard, we're headed into rougher waters.

The energies generated by the second force fuel a feisty determination to continue doing what I am doing forever. The tension created inside me by the contradictions is another source of energy and learning. I have always known I learn my most lasting lessons about difference by closely attending the ways in which the differences inside me lie down together.

November 11, 1986, New York City

I keep observing how other people die, comparing, learning, critiquing the process inside of me, matching it up to how I would like to do it. And I think about this scrutiny of myself in the context of its usefulness to other Black women living with cancer, born and unborn.

I have a privileged life or else I would be dead by now. It is two and a half years since the first tumor in my liver was discovered. When I needed to know, there was no one around to tell me that there were alternatives to turning myself over to doctors who are terrified of not knowing everything. There was no one around to remind me that I have a right to decide what happens to my own body, not because I know more than anybody else, but simply because it is my body. And I have a right to acquire the information that can help me make those crucial decisions.

It was an accident of circumstance that brought me to Germany at a critical moment in my health, and another which introduced me to one holistic/homeopathic approach to the treatment of certain cancers. Not all homeopathic alternatives work for every patient. Time is a crucial element in the treatment of cancer, and I had to decide which chances I would take, and why.

I think of what this means to other Black women living with cancer, to all women in general. Most of all I think of how important it is for us to share with each other the powers buried within the breaking of silence about our bodies and our health, even though we have been schooled to be secret and stoical about pain and disease. But that stoicism and silence does not serve us nor our communities, only the forces of things as they are.

November 12, 1986, New York City

When I write my own Book of the Dead, my own Book of Life, I want to celebrate being alive to do it even while I acknowledge the painful savor uncertainty lends to my living. I use the energy of dreams that are now impossible, not totally believing in them nor their power to become real, but recognizing them as templates for a future within which my labors can play a part. I am freer to choose what I will devote my energies toward and what I will leave for another lifetime, thanking the goddess for the strength to perceive that I can choose, despite obstacles.

So when I do a SISA reading to raise funds for the women's collectives in Soweto, or to raise money for Kitchen Table: Women of Color Press, I am choosing to use myself for things in which I passionately believe. When I speak to rally support in the urgent war against apartheid in South Africa and the racial slaughter that is even now spreading across the United States, when I demand justice in the police shotgun killing of a Black grandmother and lynchings in Northern California and in Central Park in New York City, I am making a choice of how I wish to use my power. This work gives me a tremendous amount of energy back in satisfaction and in belief, as well as in a vision of how I want this earth to be for the people who come after me.

When I work with young poets who are reaching for the power of their poetry within themselves and the lives they choose to live, I feel I am working to capacity, and this gives me deep joy, a reservoir of strength I draw upon for the next venture. Right now. This makes it far less important that it will not be forever. It never was.

The energies I gain from my work help me neutralize those implanted forces of negativity and self-destructiveness that is america's way of making sure I keep whatever is powerful and creative within me unavailable, ineffective, and nonthreatening.

But there is a terrible clarity that comes from living with cancer that can be empowering if we do not turn aside from it. What more can they do to me? My time is limited, and this is so for each one of us. So how will the opposition reward me for my silences? For the pretense that this is in fact the best of all possible worlds? What will they give me for lying? A lifelong Safe-Conduct Pass for everyone I love? Another lifetime for me? The end to racism? Sexism? Homophobia? Cruelty? The common cold?

November 13, 1986, New York City

I do not find it useful any longer to speculate upon cancer as a political weapon. But I'm not being paranoid when I say my cancer is as political as if some CIA agent brushed past me in the A train on March 15, 1965 and air-injected me with a long-fused cancer virus. Or even if it is only that I stood in their wind to do my work and the billows flayed me. What possible choices do most of us have in the air we breathe and the water we must drink?

Sometimes we are blessed with being able to choose the time and the arena and the manner of our revolution, but more usually we must do battle wherever we are standing. It does not matter too much if it is in the radiation lab or a doctor's office or the telephone company, the streets, the welfare department, or the classroom. The real blessing is to be able to use whoever I am wherever I am, in concert with as many others as possible, or alone if needs be.

This is no longer a time of waiting. It is a time for the real work's urgencies. It is a time enhanced by an iron reclamation of what I call the burst of light—that inescapable knowledge, in the bone, of my own physical limitation. Metabolized and integrated into the fabric of my days, that knowledge makes the particulars of what is coming seem less important. When I speak of wanting as much good time as possible, I mean time over which I maintain some relative measure of control.

November 14, 1986, New York City

One reason I watch the death process so acutely is to rob it of some of its power over my consciousness. I have overcome my earlier need to ignore or turn away from films and books that deal with cancer or dying. It is ever so much more important now for me to fill the psyches of all the people I love and who love me with a sense of outrageous beauty and strength of purpose.

But it is also true that sometimes we cannot heal ourselves

close to the very people from whom we draw strength and light, because they are also close to the places and tastes and smells that go along with a pattern of living we are trying to rearrange. After my mastectomy, changing the ways I ate and struggled and slept and meditated also required that I change the external environment within which I was deciding what direction I would have to take.

I am on the cusp of change and the curve is shifting fast. If any of my decisions have been in error, I must stand—not prepared, for that is impossible—but open to dealing with the consequences of those errors.

Inside and outside, change is not easy nor quick, and I find myself always on guard against what is oversimplified, or merely cosmetic.

November 15, 1986, New York City

In my office at home I have created a space that is very special to me. It is simple and quiet, with beautiful things about, and a ray of sunlight cascading through a low window on the best of days. It is here that I write whenever I am home, and where I retreat to center myself, to rest and recharge at regular intervals. It is here that I do my morning visualizations and my eurhythmics.

It is a tiny alcove with an air mattress half-covered with bright pillows, and a low narrow table with a Nigerian tie-dye throw. Against one wall and central to this space is a painting by a young Guyanese woman called *The Yard*. It is a place of water and fire and flowers and trees, filled with Caribbean women and children working and playing and being.

When the sun lances through my small window and touches the painting, the yard comes alive. The red spirit who lives at the center of the painting flames. Children laugh, a woman nurses her baby, a little naked boy cuts the grass. One woman is building a fire outside for cooking; inside a house another woman is fixing a light. In a slat-house up the hill, windows are glowing under the red-tiled roof.

I keep company with the women of this place.

Yesterday, I sat in this space with a sharp Black woman, discussing the focus of a proposed piece for a Black women's magazine. We talked about whether it should be about the role of art and spirituality in Black women's lives, or about my survival struggles with current bouts of cancer. As we talked, I gradually realized that both articles were grounded in the same place within me, and required the same focus. I require the nourishment of art and spirituality in my life, and they lend strength and insight to all the endeavors that give substance to my living. It is the bread of art and the water of my spiritual life that remind me always to reach for what is highest within my capacities and in my demands of myself and others. Not for what is perfect but for what is the best possible. And I orchestrate my daily anticancer campaign with an intensity intrinsic to who I am, the intensity of making a poem. It is the same intensity with which I experience poetry, a student's first breakthrough, the loving energy of women I do not even know, the posted photograph of a sunrise taken from my winter dawn window, the intensity of loving.

I revel in the beauty of the faces of Black women at labor and at rest. I make, demand, translate satisfactions out of every ray of sunlight, scrap of bright cloth, beautiful sound, delicious smell that comes my way, out of every sincere smile and good wish. They are discreet bits of ammunition in my arsenal against despair. They all contribute to the strengthening of my determination to persevere when the greyness overwhelms, or Reaganomics wears me down. They whisper to me of joy when the light is dim, when I falter, when another Black child is gunned down from behind in Crossroads or Newark or lynched from a tree in Memphis, and when the health orchestration gets boring or depressing or just plain too much.

November 16, 1986, New York City

For Black women, learning to consciously extend ourselves to each other and to call upon each other's strengths is a life-saving strategy. In the best of circumstances surrounding our lives, it requires an enormous amount of mutual, consistent support for us to be emotionally able to look straight into the face of the powers aligned against us and still do our work with joy.

It takes determination and practice.

Black women who survive have a head start in learning how to be open and self-protective at the same time. One secret is to ask as many people as possible for help, depending on all of them and on none of them at the same time. Some will help, others cannot. For the time being.

Another secret is to find some particular thing your soul craves for nourishment—a different religion, a quiet spot, a dance class—and satisfy it. That satisfaction does not have to be costly or difficult. Only a need that is recognized, articulated, and answered.

There is an important difference between openness and naiveté. Not everyone has good intentions nor means me well. I remind myself I do not need to change these people, only recognize who they are.

November 17, 1986, New York City

How has everyday living changed for me with the advent of a second cancer? I move through a terrible and invigorating savor of now—a visceral awareness of the passage of time, with its nightmare and its energy. No more long-term loans, extended payments, twenty-year plans. Pay my debts. Call the tickets in, the charges, the emotional IOU's. Now is the time, if ever, once and for all, to alter the patterns of isolation. Remember that nice lady down the street whose son you used to cross at the light and who was always saying, "Now if there's ever anything I can do for you, just let me know." Well, her boy's got strong muscles and the lawn needs mowing.

I am not ashamed to let my friends know I need their collective spirit—not to make me live forever, but rather to help me move through the life I have. But I refuse to spend the rest of that life mourning what I do not have.

If living as a poet—living on the front lines—has ever had meaning, it has meaning now. Living a self-conscious life, vulnerability as armor.

I spend time every day meditating upon my physical self in battle, visualizing the actual war going on inside my body. As I move through the other parts of each day, that battle often merges with particular external campaigns, both political and personal. The devastations of apartheid in South Africa and racial murder in Howard Beach feel as critical to me as cancer.

Among my other daily activities I incorporate brief periods of physical self-monitoring without hysteria. I attend the changes within my body, anointing myself with healing light. Sometimes I have to do it while sitting on the Staten Island Ferry on my way home, surrounded by snapping gum and dirty rubber boots, all of which I banish from my consciousness.

I am learning to reduce stress in my practical everyday living. It's nonsense, however, to believe that any Black woman who is living an informed life in america can possibly abolish stress totally from her life without becoming psychically deaf, mute, and blind. (News Item: Unidentified Black man found hanging from a tree in Central Park with hands and feet bound. New York City police call it a suicide.) I am learning to balance stress with periods of rest and restoration.

I juggle the technologies of eastern medicine with the holistic approach of anthroposophy with the richness of my psychic life, beautifully and womanfully nourished by people I love and who love me. Balancing them all. Knowing over and over again how blessed I am in my life, my loves, my children; how blessed I am in being able to give myself to work in which I passionately believe. And yes, some days I wish to heaven to Mawu to Seboulisa to Tiamat daughter of chaos that it could all have been easier.

But I wake in an early morning to see the sun rise over the tenements of Brooklyn across the bay, fingering through the wintered arms of the raintree Frances and I planted as a thin stick seventeen years ago, and I cannot possibly imagine trading my life for anyone else's, no matter how near termination that life may be. Living fully—how long is not the point. How and why take total precedence.

Resources on Women and Cancer

A recent article appearing in the *New England Journal of Medicine* indicated that soon after the year 2000—now less than a decade away—cancer will be the leading cause of death in the United States.* The article goes on to equivocate about the origins and prevention of cancer, completely ignoring economic, social, and environmental factors in typical mainstream medical-journal fashion, making it quite clear that the relentless increase in cancer will not be checked by those who currently reap fabulous profits from it. It's up to us.

So, where can people go if they want to work toward at least arresting the rising cancer rate? All of us, those of us who have the disease and those who have so far escaped, can throw our energies into the environmental movement. Greenpeace, for instance, has done much more to inform and educate people about the real causes of cancer than the American Cancer Society has ever done. The national office of Greenpeace is at 1436 U Street, NW, Washington, DC 20009 (202-462-1177). The national office of Citizen's Clearing House for Hazardous Wastes, Inc., another organization which is working against the increasing pollution of our environment, is P.O. Box 926, Arlington, VA 22216 (703-276-7070). And there is the National Association of Radiation Survivors, reachable at P.O. Box 20749, Oakland, CA 94620 (1-800-798-5102). There are many, many more groups of people dedicated to stemming the proliferation of poisons which cause cancer.

But many of us will want a more direct connection with the fight specifically against cancer. Literally hundreds—maybe thousands—of cancer organizations exist. Most of the groups are designed to provide emotional support or information about alternative medical services to people who have or have had cancer, or to the family, lovers, and friends of people with cancer. John Fink put together a very useful encyclopedia of these groups in *Third Opinion, An International Directory to Alternative Therapy Centers for the Treatment and Prevention of Cancer*, published in

* Meyskens, Frank L. Jr, M.D., "Coming of Age—The Chemoprevention of Cancer," *The New England Journal of Medicine*, Sept. 20, 1990, pp. 825-826.

1988 by Avery Publishing Group in Garden City, New York. I got the book by writing Project CURE, 2020 K Street, NW., Suite 350, Washington DC 20069 (1-800-552-CURE). This group recently publiished *Repression and Reform in the Evaluation of Alternative Cancer Therapies* by Robert Houston, a well-known science writer who has been an outspoken advocate for alternative approaches to the treatment of cancer.

Since breast cancer is a leading cancer-killer among women in the United States (a fact reflected in the preponderance of breast cancer represented in this anthology), there are many cancer organizations dedicated to the fight against breast cancer exclusively. The National Alliance of Breast Cancer Organizations is a good source for locating groups which limit their scope to breast cancer. Their address: NABCO, 2nd Floor, 1180 Avenue of the Americas, New York, NY 10036 (212-719-0154). They publish a newsletter, the subscription price for which is $25 per year.

There are also some organizations which not only provide support and services for people with cancer, but which additionally do research and education about the politics of cancer. I hesitate to list the groups I know only because I also know I am leaving out the many more I don't know about, so this list is to be considered just an introduction. I found out about all sorts of organizations and publications by contacting the several I knew, and each connection brought me information about others. Women who do not live on either coast of the United States or near Chicago can start by contacting any of the following organizations, and from them they may well learn of others nearer to where they live:

Breast Cancer Action
P.O. Box 460185
San Francisco, CA 94146
(415-922-8279 or 285-3626)

Cancer Support Community
401 Laurel
San Francisco, CA 94118
(415-929-7400)

Lesbian Community Cancer Project
2524 No. Lincoln Avenue, Apt. 199
Chicago, IL 60614
(312-549-4729)

The Mautner Project for Lesbians with Cancer
P.O. Box 90437
Washington, DC 20090
(202-332-5536)

Women's Cancer Resource Center
3023 Shattuck Avenue
Berkeley, CA 94705
(415-548-WCRC)

Women's Community Cancer Project
c/o The Women's Center
46 Pleasant Street
Cambridge, MA 02139
(617-354-9888)

There are many organizations dedicated to working on women's general health issues which, of course, also deal with cancer. Here are just two:

National Women's Health Network
1325 G Street, NW
Washington, DC 20005
(202-347-1140)

Black Women's Health Project
1237 Gordon Street, SW
Atlanta, GA 30310
(404-681-4554)

There may be other such libraries established to give nonmedical people access to medical information, but the one I know about is PlaneTree, 2040 Webster Street, San Francisco, CA 94115 (415-923-3680); for a fee, PlaneTree will assemble and mail a packet of the latest articles published from mainstream and alternative sources on any particular health question. Another source of more orthodox information and referrals is the national cancer hotline in Denver, Colorado: 1-800-525-3777. No one searching for more material should overlook the references cited by many of the authors in this book; they provide a rich source of information.

Lastly, there are many very good regular publications which provide ongoing news about cancer, the controversies, the research, the politics, and where to find out more. A few of the ones I have found most helpful are:

The Cancer Chronicles ($20/year)
161 West 61st Street
New York, NY 10023

Rachel's Hazardous Waste News (weekly; $40/year)
Environmental Research Foundation
P.O. Box 73700
Washington, DC 20056-3700

Science for the People ($18/year)
Science Resource Center
897 Main Street
Cambridge, MA 02139

The most hopeful and encouraging aspect to this list of resources is the fact that thousands of groups do not appear, not because they are unimportant, but simply because there are too many organizations to list. No one, however, should assume that her help is not needed because there are already so many groups; a successful battle against the proliferation of cancer will require still many, many more of us. Nonetheless, all of these organizations do mean that with very little effort any woman can find a source of information and support or a place to work where her energies can go to making our country and our planet a healthy place once again in which to live, a place where someday cancer will no longer invade the bodies of one in three people.

Judith Brady, Editor
April, 1991

About the Authors

Sharon Batt lives in Montréal, Québec where she is a writer and a researcher. She was diagnosed with breast cancer in November of 1988.

June Beisch, a Minnesota-born poet, teaches American literature at Massachusetts Bay Community College in Wellesley. Her poetry and reviews have been published in several literary journals. She worked for ten years as a free-lance writer for *The Boston Globe*, and she has been a recipient of the Middlesex County Poetry Award, sponsored by *Atlantic Monthly*.

Elizabeth Brunazzi grew up in Louisiana and East Texas. Her poetry and fiction have previously appeared in the *Washington Review, off our backs* and several anthologies. She currently lives in New York City and teaches in the Department of Romance Languages at Wesleyan University in Middletown, Connecticut. She recently received a Camargo Foundation grant for 1991 to write a book on images of women in history, film, and literature during the Nazi Occupation of France.

Nancy Bruning writes about health, fitness, medicine, and the environment. She is the author or co-author of eight books; her work has also appeared in many magazines, newspapers, and patient-information booklets. Her diagnosis of breast cancer in 1981 prompted her to write *Coping with Chemotherapy* (Ballantine Books, 1985), a guideline for patients with all types of cancer.

Lois Camp is a farm wife living in LaCrosse, Washington. Her love of the rural life lies behind her efforts to preserve and protect the heritage and the land of her community. She continues to be active in the efforts of Hanford Downwinders to bring the horrors of the secret Hanford radioactive emissions to the attention of the rest of the world.

Noelle Caskey recently completed an interdisciplinary doctorate at the University of California by writing a dissertation on the psychology of women writers. She has published poetry, journalism, and a scholarly article on anorexia nervosa. In addition to co-leading a support group for women with cancer at the Women's Cancer Resource Center, she serves as Associate Director of the California Humanities Project.

Helene Davis, born in Washington, D.C., grew up in Rhode Island and is currently living in Cambridge, where she teaches at the University of Massachusetts at Boston. Her poems about her cancer experience, *Chemo-Poet and Other Poems*, were published by Alice James Books in Cambridge, Massachusetts in 1989.

Rosylin Dean lives in San Jose, California, where she is involved with her community in educational, social, and political activities. Since her breast cancer at the age of 51, she has enjoyed good health and energy, which she puts to work in her union and in trying to change U.S. foreign policy in Central America, all the while keeping in mind the connections between herself and the ecological environment of Planet Earth.

Frédérique Delacoste began Cleis Press in 1980 with Felice Newman. She co-edited *Sex Work: Writings by Women in the Sex Industry* and *Fight Back! Feminist Resistance to Male Violence*.

Claude Delventhal was born in 1945 in Grenoble, France. She moved to San Francisco in 1969, where she lived until her death in 1990. She was diagnosed with breast cancer in 1981, and was very actively involved in determining her course of treatment throughout her illness, always ready to question the medical establishment. From the first, Claude was "out" as a cancer patient, and shared her life with simplicity and generosity.

Reina Diaz lives in Mountain View, California, in a small house always filled with family and friends. She remains active in her community and the never-ending struggle for justice for all people.

Susan Eisenberg is a poet/writer, mother, and union electrician living in Boston. She is the author of several plays, articles, and the poetry book, *It's a Good Thing I'm Not Macho* (Whetstone Press, 1984). Under a grant from the Witter Bynner Foundation for Poetry, she recently developed *Coffee Break Secrets*, a performance piece and video scripted from poems about daily work.

Zinna Epperson lives in Shingletown, California. An Arcona/Cherokee mixed blood Native American, she is disabled with systemic lupus and is, so far, a Hanford radiation survivor. She has four living children. Due to growing physical limitations, Zinna now concentrates mostly on art and writing.

Janis Coombs Epps is currently Associate Academic Dean at DeKalb College's central campus in Atlanta, Georgia. She is the mother of two children who keep her busily involved in their activities. She is an avid reader, family historian, and free-lance writer.

Adele Friedman, once chair of the Department of Liberal Arts of the National Technical Institute for the Deaf/Rochester Institute of Technology, and former Professor of French in the California State University system, was active in cancer support groups, the Eco-Justice Network, and the Center for Independent Living in Rochester, New York. Adele died from cancer in the spring of 1991.

Lisa Gayle is a writer and a high school science teacher. She is completing a novel about women working in an auto plant. She lives with her husband, Michael, and their young son in Detroit.

Carol Givens, determined to have a life different from that of her childhood in Detroit, joined the Air Force as a way of securing her education. She married, divorced, and discovered that her deepest love was for women. She moved with her lover to Sonoma County, California in 1984, the same year she discovered her cancer. Carol died on January 12, 1989, after saying goodbye to all her friends.

Barbara Hoffman lives in New York State and has published in *Beloit Poetry Journal*, *Gryphon*, and *Aura/Literary Arts Journal*. She has appeared on radio and television, and has been a Poetry Workshop leader at Suffolk County Prison facilities in Yaphank and Riverhead, New York.

Karen Hopkins is forty years old, and lives in Albany, California with her two sons. After her thyroid cancer, she changed jobs to a "regular" eight-to-five office position in order to reduce stress in her life—the nineties answer for good health.

April Lindner lives in Yonkers, New York, and recently earned a Master of Fine Arts in Writing from Sarah Lawrence College. Her poems have been published in numerous publications.

Susan Liroff is a forty-four-year-old Jewish lesbian who spent twenty years being a vegetarian. She also used to be a fitness fanatic. She was very surprised when she found out that she had cancer.

Simi Litvak grew up in Denver, Colorado, sixteen miles from Rocky Flats. A survivor of thyroid and breast cancer and a long-time activist in the progressive women's movement, she now lives in Oakland, California where she is a research director of the World Institute on Disability and the Research and Training Center on Public Policy in Independent Living.

Audre Lorde is a Black lesbian warrior poet now living in the Virgin Islands. She is also a teacher, a political activist, and a mother. Among her many books are two pioneering chronicles of her personal and political struggles with cancer: *The Cancer Journals* (Aunt Lute Books, San Francisco, 1980) and *A Burst of Light* (Firebrand Books, Ithaca, New York, 1988). Her powerful voice has lent its strength and her passion for survival to multitudes of women.

Jackie Manthorne is a writer, editor and publisher living in Montréal, Québec. Her work has appeared in several anthologies, including *By Word of Mouth: Lesbians Write the Erotic* (Gynergy Books) and *The Guide to Gracious Lesbian Living* (Lilith Publications), as well as in periodicals.

Marsha Caddell Mathews' poetry appears in the *Kansas Quarterly* and *North of Wakulla: An Anhinga Anthology*. Her play, *The Darkest Hour*, has been produced at State Street Methodist Church in Bristol, Virginia. She has a collection of poems, *The Rise Above the Water*, and is working on another, *Prophet on a Wing*.

Nicola Morris teaches feminist studies, writing and literature at Goddard College in Plainfield, Vermont. She has published poems, stories, and essays in feminist journals.

Holly O. is in her early twenties. She lives in Kansas City and works as a writer for a national magazine. When not writing, she reads and spends time with her family and friends.

Sandy Polishuk has been a radio programmer, textile artist, and political activist. She is a member of the Northwest Women's History Project, producer of the slide show, "Good Work Sisters," an oral history of women shipyard workers during World War II. She is currently working on oral histories of political activists and of breast cancer survivors.

Nita Rabinovitch lives part of the year in Norman, Oklahoma, where she was Director of Social Work Services at the Norman Regional Hospital until 1987, when she resigned to write and concentrate on healing. She also lives part of the year in Vermont, where she can be near her daughters and grandsons, and where she sells vegetables and flowers at the Farmer's Market.

Linda Reyes is a native of the San Francisco Bay Area, where she has lived all her life and raised her five children. She's been battling cancer for more than a decade, and the two San Francisco organizations in which she is an active member, Breast Cancer Action and the Cancer Support Community, keep her in touch with reality and provide her with vehicles through which to expose cancer not just as a personal tragedy, but as a major social/economic problem.

Ines Rieder, co-editor of *AIDS: The Women* (Cleis Press, 1988) and *Cosmopolis: Urban Stories by Women* (Cleis Press, 1990), grew up in a family of doctors in Vienna. That's where she learned not only to advocate patients' rights, but also to understand the necessity of a public health care system which takes care of everyone, regardless of their class background.

Barbara Rosenblum was born on April 9, 1943 and died on February 14, 1988. During her forty-four years, she was a teacher both at Stanford University and Goddard College; a writer of articles both scholarly and personal; involved in community both artistic and political, and a loving partner to Sandra Butler, with whom she wrote *Cancer in Two Voices*. Her essays on the political meanings of breast cancer are the genesis of the piece in this volume.

Beverly Ross is a civil servant who works and lives in the Washington, D.C. area. Her medical prognosis is excellent. She and Linda are planning their lives together.

Mary Ryan has been active in the Mautner Project in Washington, D.C. since the first community meeting in 1990. Her partner died of breast cancer.

Anna Shaler has survived two bouts with breast cancer, feels great, and considers this next part of her life to be gravy. She's had a career as a dancer and as an actress, has written a novel, and lives in New York City with her daughter. She is currently at work on a collection of short stories.

Deborah Smith was a Phi Beta Kappa graduate of the University of California at Berkeley, and received her master's in economics from the Davis campus. Since 1986 she served as Vice President of Planning and Corporate Development for the Chase Manhattan Bank in New York while living with her husband in Sparta, New Jersey. Deborah died on February 19, 1990 after a seventeen-month battle against leukemia.

Millie Smith, who grew up in Pasco, Washington near the Hanford Nuclear Site, now lives in Olympia, Washington. She describes herself as an American Hibakusha, and she spends what time and energy she has in the struggle to help radiation victims worldwide and to stop further contamination of our planet.

Sandra Steingraber teaches biology and science writing at Columbia College in Chicago and researches environmental human rights issues. She is co-author of the book, *Spoils of Famine: Ethiopian Famine Policy and Peasant Agriculture*. She has completed a poetry manuscript, *Post-Diagnosis*.

Jackie Winnow, a forty-three-year-old transplanted New Yorker living in Oakland, California, is the founder of the Women's Cancer Resource Center in Berkeley. She was the Coordinator of the Lesbian/Gay and AIDS Unit of the San Francisco Human Rights Commission. She is a cancer activist, lesbian feminist, cat aficionada, haggler for social justice, and a lover of life. She has metastatic breast cancer of the lungs and bones; no moment passes without the awareness of cancer and the need to learn to adjust to an ever changing and limiting body.

Cindy Winslow arrived in San Francisco by motorcycle in 1973 and ten years later went to Mexico to write an autobiography and run the English department of a Mexican high school. She returned to San Francisco in 1987 and faced cancer in 1988. She is now working as a state government analyst dealing with the issues of health care and the elderly, and she is also the treasurer of the Women's Cancer Resource Center in Berkeley, California.

About the Editor

Judith Brady, who earns her living as a secretary, is a long-time activist in progressive movements; her political birth came through the women's liberation movement of the late 1960s. She is the author of the now-classic essay, "Why I Want A Wife," first published in the premier issue of *Ms*. Magazine in the spring of 1972 (reprinted as "Why I [Still] Want a Wife," *Ms. Magazine*, July/August, 1990). The ideological understanding of the connection between the personal and the political, which she learned as a feminist, underlies her conviction that her private experience with cancer has a political genesis, and this book is the result.

Books from Cleis Press

Recommended Health/Recovery Titles:

The Absence of the Dead Is Their Way of Appearing by Mary Winfrey Trautmann. ISBN: 0-939416-04-2 8.95 paper.

AIDS: The Women edited by Ines Rieder and Patricia Ruppelt. ISBN: 0-939416-20-4 24.95 cloth; ISBN: 0-939416-21-2 9.95 paper.

Don't: A Woman's Word by Elly Danica. ISBN: 0-939416-23-9 21.95 cloth; ISBN: 0-939416-22-0 8.95 paper.

1 in 3: Women with Cancer Confront an Epidemic edited by Judith Brady. ISBN: 0-939416-50-6 24.95 cloth; ISBN: 0-939416-49-2 10.95 paper.

Voices in the Night: Women Speaking About Incest edited by Toni A.H. McNaron and Yarrow Morgan. ISBN: 0-939416-02-6 9.95 paper.

With the Power of Each Breath: A Disabled Women's Anthology edited by Susan Browne, Debra Connors and Nanci Stern. ISBN: 0-939416-09-3 24.95 cloth; ISBN: 0-939416-06-9 10.95 paper.

Woman-Centered Pregnancy and Birth by the Federation of Feminist Women's Health Centers. ISBN: 0-939416-03-4 11.95 paper.

Women's Studies

Peggy Deery: An Irish Family at War by Nell McCafferty. ISBN: 0-939416-38-7 24.95 cloth; ISBN: 0-939416-39-5 9.95 paper.

Sex Work: Writings by Women in the Sex Industry edited by Frédérique Delacoste and Priscilla Alexander. ISBN: 0-939416-10-7 24.95 cloth; ISBN: 0-939416-11-5 12.95 paper.

The Shape of Red: Insider/Outsider Reflections by Ruth Hubbard and Margaret Randall. ISBN: 0-939416-19-0 24.95 cloth; ISBN: 0-939416-18-2 9.95 paper.

Women & Honor: Some Notes on Lying by Adrienne Rich. ISBN: 0-939416-44-1 3.95 paper.

Animal Rights

And a Deer's Ear, Eagle's Song and Bear's Grace: Relationships Between Animals and Women edited by Theresa Corrigan and Stephanie T. Hoppe. ISBN: 0-939416-38-7 24.95 cloth; ISBN: 0-939416-39-5 9.95 paper.

With a Fly's Eye, Whale's Wit and Woman's Heart: Relationships Between Animals and Women edited by Theresa Corrigan and Stephanie T. Hoppe. ISBN: 0-939416-24-7 24.95 cloth; ISBN: 0-939416-25-5 9.95 paper.

Fiction

Another Love by Erzsébet Galgóczi. ISBN: 0-939416-52-2 24.95 cloth; ISBN: 0-939416-51-4 8.95 paper.

Cosmopolis: Urban Stories by Women edited by Ines Rieder. ISBN: 0-939416-36-0 24.95 cloth; ISBN: 0-939416-37-9 9.95 paper.

Night Train To Mother by Ronit Lentin. ISBN: 0-939416-29-8 24.95 cloth; ISBN: 0-939416-28-X 9.95 paper.

The One You Call Sister: New Women's Fiction edited by Paula Martinac. ISBN: 0-939416-30-1 24.95 cloth; ISBN: 0-939416031-X 9.95 paper.

Unholy Alliances: New Women's Fiction edited by Louise Rafkin. ISBN: 0-939416-14-X 21.95 cloth; ISBN: 0-939416-15-8 9.95 paper.

The Wall by Marlen Haushofer. ISBN: 0-939416-53-0 24.95 cloth; ISBN: 0-939416-54-9 paper.

Latin American Studies

Beyond the Border: A New Age in Latin American Women's Fiction edited by Nora Erro-Peralta and Caridad Silva-Núñez. ISBN: 0-939416-42-5 24.95 cloth; ISBN: 0-939416-43-3 12.95 paper.

The Little School: Tales of Disappearance and Survival in Argentina by Alicia Partnoy. ISBN: 0-939416-08-5 21.95 cloth; ISBN: 0-939416-07-7 9.95 paper.

You Can't Drown the Fire: Latin American Women Writing in Exile edited by Alicia Partnoy. ISBN: 0-939416-16-6 24.95 cloth; ISBN: 0-939416-17-4 9.95 paper.

Lesbian Studies

A Lesbian Love Advisor by Celeste West. ISBN: 0-939416-27-1 24.95 cloth; ISBN: 0-939416-26-3 9.95 paper.

Different Daughters: A Book by Mothers of Lesbians edited by Louise Rafkin. ISBN: 0-939416-12-3 21.95 cloth; ISBN: 0-939416-13-1 9.95 paper.

Different Mothers: Sons & Daughters of Lesbians Talk About Their Lives edited by Louise Rafkin. ISBN: 0-939416-40-9 24.95 cloth; ISBN: 0-939416-41-7 9.95 paper.

Long Way Home: The Odyssey of a Lesbian Mother and Her Children by Jeanne Jullion. ISBN: 0-939416-05-0 8.95 paper.

More Serious Pleasure: Lesbian Erotic Stories and Poetry edited by the Sheba Collective. ISBN: 0-939416-48-4 24.95 cloth; ISBN: 0-939416-47-6 9.95 paper.

Serious Pleasure: Lesbian Erotic Stories and Poetry edited by the Sheba Collective. ISBN: 0-939416-46-8 24.95 cloth; ISBN: 0-939416-45-X 9.95 paper.

Susie Sexpert's Lesbian Sex World by Susie Bright. ISBN: 0-939416-34-4 24.95 cloth; ISBN: 0-939416-35-2 9.95 paper.

Since 1980, Cleis Press has published progressive books by women. We welcome your order and will ship your books as quickly as possible. Individual orders must be prepaid (U.S. dollars only). Please add 15% shipping. PA residents add 6% sales tax. Mail orders: Cleis Press, PO Box 8933, Pittsburgh PA 15221. MasterCard and Visa orders: $25 minimum—include account number, exp. date, and signature. FAX your credit card order: (412) 937-1567. Or, phone us Mon-Fri, 9 am - 5 pm EST: (412) 937-1555.